D0443070

# THE ORIENTAL
# 7-DAY QUICK WEIGHT-OFF DIET

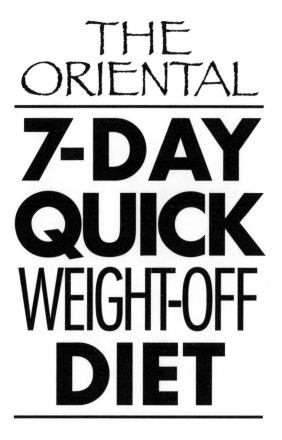

NORVELL

Revised by

JOHN HEINERMAN

PRENTICE HALL

**Library of Congress Cataloging-in-Publication Data**

Norvell.
    The oriental 7-day quick weight-off diet / by Anthony Norvell ;
revised and updated by John Heinerman. — Rev. ed.
      p.   cm.
    Includes index.
    ISBN 0-13-254905-0 (cloth)—ISBN 0-13-254913-1 (paper)
    1. Reducing diets—Recipes.   2. Cookery, Oriental.   I. Heinerman,
John.  II. Title.
RM222.2.N67   1996                               96-11255
613.2′5—dc20                                       CIP

© *1996 by Prentice-Hall, Inc.*

*All rights reserved. No part of this book may be reproduced in any form or by any means, without permission in writing from the publisher.*

*Printed in the United States of America*

*10   9   8            (cloth)*

*10   9   8   7   6   5   4   3   2   1   (paper)*

This book is a reference work based on research by the author. The opinions expressed herein are not necessarily those of or endorsed by the publisher. The directions stated in this book are in no way to be considered as a substitute for consultation with a duly licensed doctor.

ISBN 0-13-254905-0 (cloth)

ISBN 0-13-254913-1 (paper)

---

**ATTENTION: CORPORATIONS AND SCHOOLS**

Prentice Hall books are available at quantity discounts with bulk purchase for educational, business, or sales promotional use. For information, please write to: Prentice Hall Special Sales, 240 Frisch Court, Paramus, New Jersey 07652. Please supply: title of book, ISBN number, quantity, how the book will be used, date needed.

---

**PRENTICE HALL**
**Paramus, NJ 07652**

On the World Wide Web at http://www.phdirect.com

*Dedicated to my many wonderful friends at*
*Wakunaga of America:*

Mitsuru Takiura

George Tsutsuse

Charlie Fox

Bill Sterling

Jay Levy

# Also by the Author

*Norvell's Dynamic Mental Laws for Successful Living* (1965)

*Meta-Physics: New Dimensions of the Mind* (1967)

*Cosmic Magnetism: The Miracle of the Magic Power Circle* (1970)

*Mind Cosmology* (1971)

*Occult Sciences: How to Get What You Want Through Your Occult Powers* (1971)

*The Miracle Power of Transcendental Meditation* (1972)

*One Hundred Thousand Dollar Dream and How to Make It Come True* (1973)

*Universal Secrets of Telecosmic Power* (1974)

# Also by Dr. Heinerman

*Heinerman's Encyclopedia of Fruits, Vegetables and Herbs* (1988)

*Double the Power of Your Immune System* (1991)

*Heinerman's Encyclopedia of Healing Juices* (1994)

*Heinerman's Encyclopedia of Nuts, Berries and Seeds* (1995)

*Heinerman's Encyclopedia of Fruits and Vegetables* (revised edition, 1995)

*Heinerman's Encyclopedia of Healing Herbs and Spices* (1995)

*Heinerman's Encyclopedia of Juices, Teas and Tonics* (1996)

*Heinerman's Encyclopedia of Anti-Aging* (1996)

# FOREWORD TO THIS EDITION

Over two decades ago, Anthony Norvell came out with this book bearing the quirky title *The Oriental 7-Day Quick Weight-Off Diet*. Right away the book took off, almost overnight becoming a bestseller. So successful has it been that twenty-two years later it still remains in print. The single reason for its publishing longevity is that *the diet really works!* In an era where the average shelf life of a book is usually no more than one year in hardback and one or two years in paperback, this slim volume has outlived Pulitzer Prize–winning books and famous novels from which big-screen movies or television shows have been made.

The late Mr. Norvell wasn't a doctor or even a trained scientist. He was just an ordinary fellow writing for the layperson. But through his investigative work, reading, experimentation, and thinking he came up with this "quick weight-off diet" that can be done in a week or ten days if you put your mind and heart to it.

Like anything else in life, it takes a certain amount of work and effort to realize something you may want very much. And who doesn't want to be more slender and beautiful anyway? Obesity has been ranked by the American medical profession as "a national disease," not to mention being a national disgrace.

Mr. Norvell wrote his book at a time when the thinking about nutritional and health matters was a lot different than it is now. For instance, back in the 1970s, no one considered bologna or cream cheese to be detrimental to weight loss, let alone bad for the heart. Mr. Norvell occasionally recommended such things as snack foods, and made other suggestions that are now considered questionable. Consequently, some changes in the text were necessary.

This is where I came into the picture. The publisher approached me with an invitation that I couldn't resist. (This is the second book by a well-known author that I've revised. The first was

*Back to Eden* by Jethro Kloss. Members of the Kloss family employed my services in the early 1980s to update what has become America's all-time best-selling herb book.)

I have spent the better part of fifteen years of my life touring most of the countries ringing the Pacific Rim, spending considerable time in nearly every country from Taiwan and Japan to Singapore and Indonesia. I am well acquainted with the Orient, its customs and habits, languages and cultures, and diets and folk remedies. What I've tried to bring to Mr. Norvell's work is a certain scientific discipline that was lacking in the original. By this statement, I in no way wish to denigrate what Mr. Norvell himself wrote; rather I mean that a *more scientific* approach has been taken with the information I've contributed, to make our *combined* efforts more plausible and credible to readers.

Each of us felt in our own individual ways that a lot can be done about shedding unwanted pounds, looking better, and feeling great. And we felt that some of the best methods for bringing this about lie in the Orient. So while it can be said that Anthony Norvell built the house (or wrote the book), it took my efforts to reinforce the foundation thereof and make some significant changes within. The end result is *a newly remodeled house,* patterned after the old blueprints, but with a lot of new plumbing, wiring, and other fixtures to make it more livable and workable.

*The Oriental 7-Day Quick Weight-Off Diet* DID WORK for several million people in its original edition. But now it WILL WORK EVEN BETTER, thanks to what modern science has since discovered.

*John Heinerman, Ph.D.*

# INTRODUCTION

■ ■ ■

## WHY MOST PEOPLE CANNOT DIET SUCCESSFULLY

Most people hate to diet because most reducing diets deprive them of all the foods that give them pleasure. People dislike any diet plan that makes them feel perpetually hungry.

Hunger is nature's way of warning us that the body mechanism requires nourishment to sustain the life function. Subconsciously it is alarming for the person to feel hunger pangs. One's first instinct is to eat until the hunger pangs go away. This usually means eating the things that most quickly satisfy the appetite.

The foods that give stomach satisfaction and quick energy are the carbohydrate foods: starches, sugars, and fats. These satisfy hunger immediately, but they are quickly converted into stored energy or excess fat.

It is much more satisfying to the taste buds to feast on ice cream and cake than to eat proteins, grains, and vegetables, for the carbohydrates give taste satisfaction that these do not give. However, carbohydrates require the body to store the excess energy, producing fat, and soon the person is hungry once again and continues the vicious cycle of eating to satisfy his hunger pangs.

■ ■ ■

## THE 7-DAY MIRACLE DIET DOES AWAY WITH HUNGER!

The wonderful thing about the 7-day Oriental miracle diet is that it does away with hunger pangs entirely! This should be the first requirement in any adequate diet that will properly nourish the body and yet give a sense of satisfaction to the person who is trying to reduce.

A woman I once knew was unhappy in her marriage and ate her way to 210 pounds in a year's time. She could not stop eating candy and other sweets. She began to gain weight, and the more she gained the more she ate to keep up the body fat.

When she came to me for advice, she had already lost her husband's love, and he was running around with other women. Out of desperation this woman decided to try the 7-day miracle diet. The first thing she did was to establish the fact she would not be hungry during the dieting, which in her case would require several months. When she found that with this diet she could eat as much as she wanted of certain foods, she was delighted, and thus one of the most serious mental blocks was overcome.

In this woman's case, she continued to diet beyond the seven-day period, for her weight was so great that she could not lose sufficient weight in the first week. But within one year's time she was back to her normal weight of 130 pounds and not only won back her husband's love but felt better than ever before. She was then put on a sustaining diet to keep her weight at normal.

The 7-day Oriental miracle diet will give you the following benefits immediately:

1. You will be able to lose as much weight as you wish, easily and quickly, with little effort on your part and without having to starve yourself. You will be able to eat all the food you want, as much as four or five pounds a day, and you will feel constantly full and satisfied.

2. You will be given a variety of good and nourishing foods that are tasty and, without counting calories, will give you the illusion that you are constantly stuffed. This will help remove the subconscious alarm bell that rings when most people try to diet and that makes them keep eating the quick-energy-producing foods that make fat. These foods do not sustain the body's energy, failing to keep the blood sugar content at high levels, which is required for steady energy output.

3. You will be able to eat not just three square meals a day, but as many as six or eight! In other words, you will eat as often as you wish and whenever you feel hungry. This food intake will be the type that *does not* go to fat.

4. You will have a sense of well-being. This is psychologically important, for most people cannot remain on a reducing diet for any length of time, without becoming irritable and feeling a sense of nervousness, which makes them turn to food as a source of consolation.

   The foods on the 7-day miracle diet will remove that sense of irritability by making you feel full and satisfied. The resulting psychological benefits will be such that you will constantly have a sense of well-being.

5. You can eat a wide variety of foods that give you the perfect nourishment. These foods will also help satisfy your hunger urge. You can eat most lean meats, fish, eggs, cheese and other milk products, and vegetables, as well as certain types of fruits.

6. You will get proper, balanced nutrition that will make it possible for you to do a full day's work, with more energy than ever before. You will seldom feel tired and lazy, as you may when you are stuffed with the wrong types of carbohydrates, starches, and fats. The reason for this is that this diet will give you all the necessary carbohydrates, proteins, vitamins, and minerals your body requires for perfect health. This diet will not only cause you to reduce your weight to its correct level, but when you continue on the weight-sustaining diet, you will not put back on the weight that you have lost. This is the error in most quick-reducing plans!

7. You will be given a list of "negative-energizer" foods that actually help burn away the body fat. These foods will reduce your weight because they require more energy to digest than they give to the body. This means that the more of these reducing foods you eat, the more weight you will lose!

If you ate nothing for a period of ten days, you would lose only about a pound a day. But if you eat the reducing foods on the list, you will lose as much as two pounds a day! This is the secret behind the Oriental 7-day reducing diet—the more you eat of these special foods, the more you lose, for it takes more calories to digest these foods than they give to your body!

8. You will actually begin to lose from one to two pounds a day immediately. If you happen to be only ten pounds overweight, the 7-day miracle diet will be sufficient and require little effort or will power on your part.

   However, if you happen to be from twenty to fifty pounds overweight, or even more, you need not stop at the end of seven days, but you can continue for a period of three or four weeks, eating all the food you want and still burning up the body fat until you reach your required, normal weight.

9. After you have lost the pounds you want, you will then go on a sustaining diet that you will follow the rest of your life. This diet will keep you slender, give you great energy, and constantly keep you at the weight you desire.

   However, if you binge occasionally and put on a few pounds, the 7-day diet can be used again, and you will quickly lose the undesired pounds. This will remove the psychological fear that you are going to get back the lost pounds and be as fat as you were before. When you once know that you can go on a corrective diet for only a few days, you will no longer fear dieting.

10. You will be given a variety of tasty menus that are nourishing and that make you feel you are not really dieting but trying new and delicious recipes. You will learn exotic dishes from the Orient that you can add to your regular diet and that will make you a gourmet cook with little effort or expense.

11. You are *will not be* denied the fat-producing foods, which are generally more delicious than typical dieting foods. These fat-producing foods such as meat, fish, cheese, milk, and eggs furnish the body with calories that are quickly turned into fat. This is why diets that tell you to eat as much as you wish of

meat, eggs, and cheese are faulty. However, in this diet, you will learn how to mix these fat-producing foods with the weight-reducing foods, such as vegetables, grains, and fruit, and as it requires more calories to digest these foods than the body receives in energy, these foods will make you lose weight safely and quickly.

The reason this 7-day Oriental miracle diet works so beautifully is that it psychologically conditions you to the fact that it is simple to follow and that there are no mental or physical hazards. So many people find it difficult to stick to a diet because they feel it is a dreary and long-drawn-out chore that will tax them mentally and physically.

In this 7-day miracle diet we use the same principle that guides alcoholics in their fight to free themselves from drinking—they go without alcohol one day at a time, until they gain such strength that they can do without a drink for days or months.

It is easy to visualize yourself cutting down on food for a period of only one week. In fact, it is fun, for there is sufficient food intake to keep you from ever growing hungry. Then, by the end of seven days, when you see the dramatic results, your willpower is so strengthened that you can continue the 7-day diet for another seven days—or as many more as you require to get you down to your normal weight.

*Anthony Norvell*

# CONTENTS

# CHAPTER 1

# THE NATURAL ORIENTAL DIET FOR LOSING WEIGHT WITHOUT HUNGER

T hrough the natural Oriental diet, which is the basis of my 7-day diet plan to reduce without hunger, you can begin to lose weight from the very first day without any effort on your part and without the hunger pangs usually associated with dieting. Then, when you have lost your undesired pounds, you can keep your weight at a normal level through a pleasant, safe, and effortless diet that has been used by millions of people in the Far East for centuries.

On this 7-day miracle diet you can have a maximum degree of efficiency, continue your work, and enjoy a perfectly normal life. There will be no periods of weakness, depression, nervousness, headaches, or other symptoms that usually follow most efforts to reduce. This is because you can avoid the gnawing hunger pangs that usually accompany most weight-reducing diets. You do this by eating as many of the weight-reducing foods on the diet as you wish, at any time you feel hungry, and you need not fear that they will be converted into unwanted fat!

■ ■ ■

## HOW THE 7-DAY MIRACLE DIET WILL CREATE BALANCE IN YOUR LIFE

Not only is it vitally important to eat a balanced diet, even while reducing, but it is even more important that you build a mental philosophy that can keep your mind calm and controlled during your period of dieting, so you can absorb the nutrients necessary to keep the body healthy and normal during your stringent period of dieting.

To prove the importance of maintaining a high level of energy through a balanced diet even when you are reducing, an experiment was conducted by nutritionists. They put a group of ten young women on a stringent diet. The women were given overcooked vegetables from which all nutrients were removed. They were given white bread and white sugar and allowed to eat pastries, canned fruits in heavy syrup, ice cream and cake, and other heavy carbohydrate foods. All fresh vegetables and salads were eliminated from their diet, and the women were not allowed to eat any form of protein, such as meat, or cheese, or other milk products. Even eggs were prohibited.

On this restricted diet, within two weeks, these normally healthy young women became fatigued, nervous, and neurotic. They quarreled over trifles; they lost any desire to do any kind of work. The more they ate of this restricted diet, the worse they became until some of them actually seemed to be psychotic.

When these women were put back on a normal diet of fruits, vegetables and balanced proteins, they recovered from their symptoms and had their former feelings of well-being and energy without fatigue, irritability, and lassitude. Another important effect was that the tendency to overeat, which came with their predominantly carbohydrate diet, began to add pounds to their weight, and only when they returned to their normal diets did they begin to stabilize their weight.

■ ■ ■

## PROTEINS IMPORTANT IN ANY REDUCING PLAN

In my study of the diet problems of most overweight people I discovered that they ate plenty of food, but it was mostly of the wrong kind. They ate the denatured, overcooked, fattening foods that gave them bulk but were lacking in nourishment.

It is vitally important in any weight-reducing diet that there be sufficient protein to meet one's daily energy needs. This is determined by the expenditure of energy in a day's work. Obviously, a sedentary worker requires fewer calories than a laborer does. Although with the Oriental 7-day miracle diet we do not count calories, it is important to know about calories and to avoid taking in too many calories while on the reducing plan. At least sixty grams of protein daily is essential to proper nourishment.

This daily intake of protein assures the body of getting enough nourishment to supply the requirements for vitality and energy. We take into account the fact that the body requires this protein intake every day, even while reducing. This is especially true for those who are past age forty, when the body requires certain proteins and amino acids that are essential to proper nourishment. Without these amino acids, furnished by proteins, the body cannot manufacture the proper enzymes that effect metabolism and that give the body nourishment. This is why many people feel so fatigued while they are dieting.

■ ■ ■

## LOSING WEIGHT WITHOUT LOSING ENERGY

With my 7-day Oriental diet you will avoid another serious dietary deficiency—the serious drop in blood sugar that most dieters experience when they go on a drastic weight-reducing program. On this 7-day miracle diet you can eat all you want of nonfattening foods and you need never experience hunger. You may eat as often as six to eight times a day and still lose your quota of two pounds a day!

The problem with dieting for those who have been diagnosed with hypoglycemia is that any temporary fasting or meal delays cause a sudden drop in blood sugar levels. This can have a profound effect on their entire body chemistry. Immediate fatigue, unexpected drowsiness, frequent bouts of irritability, and dramatic mood swings are some of the most common symptoms.

I've designed my system so that you can actually snack throughout the day without gaining any more weight or adversely affecting your blood sugar levels, in the event that you're one of those with hypoglycemia. The secret to this snacking is the *quality* of the food consumed. I recommend lots of protein and additional amino acid supplements. Also, the person with low blood sugar intending to go on my diet should eat something every two and a half hours, if she feels her body getting weak.

And while part of my diet obviously includes a lot of fruits, which are ordinarily healthful to eat for normal individuals, they may not always be the best for hypoglycemics to snack on. If you already know you have low blood sugar, may I suggest that you focus on a wide array of vegetables, both raw and lightly cooked, instead? They will provide the body with enough energy, without dumping a lot of natural sugars into it.

I also advocate that carbohydrates be consumed in more complex arrangements. The carbohydrates in fruits are too quickly converted into blood sugar, thus resulting in a chaotic effect on someone who is hypoglycemic. But complex carbohydrates have within their structures the necessary fibers that act as "braking" mechanisms to slow down their absorption and assimilation throughout the system.

Hence, baked potatoes, pasta, whole-grain cereals and breads, and similar foods qualify for this. They can be eaten regularly in small portions as part of the snacking process that I encourage in my diet plan.

People with hypoglycemia may also do well to combine complex carbohydrates with some protein foods in the same snack meals. Hence, a sandwich made with two slices of seven-grain or whole-wheat bread with organic almond, cashew, or all-natural peanut butter would nicely meet this criterion. Another good example is a baked potato topped with yogurt and ground, hulled sunflower seeds.

■ ■ ■

## THE ORIENTAL SYSTEM OF DIETING CLEANSES THE BODY OF TOXIC POISONS

One of the reasons why the Oriental system of dieting works to reduce weight as well as to maintain perfect health afterward is that most of the foods used in the diet are fresh, vital foods—vegetables, grains, and fruits that help keep the body in a state of alkalinity and that flush out the poisons that gather in the body through toxic wastes and the heavy carbohydrate foods. This diet helps furnish the glands with the correct nutrients that will cause them to function more efficiently and to do the job for which they were intended.

Drugs should be taken only with a physician's advice. They often tend to overstimulate the glands of the endocrine system until finally these glands are no longer able to perform their function and the entire system collapses.

In some cases, eating stimulating foods, drinking too much coffee or alcohol, or filling the system with salt, sugars, starches, and other concentrated forms of highly irritating foods, gives a temporary acceleration of the entire glandular system, causing them to oversecrete and become exhausted. Then they fail in their vital functions, with fatal results.

### A Woman Suffering from Overstimulated Glands

The case came to my attention of Lillian P., a woman who was very much overweight—about fifty pounds. She suffered from severe arthritis, high blood pressure, and other ailments that kept her constantly sick. She told me she drank from eight to ten cups of coffee a day. She claimed that she needed its stimulus to keep her going during the day. Then at night, despite the fact that she was exhausted, she was so nervous and tense that she couldn't sleep. She then took sleeping pills to help her rest. Finally she was taking so many sleeping pills that they ceased to be effective. With her doctor's cooperation, I told her first to give up coffee and drink a caffeine-free substitute. Lillian went on the Oriental diet, using no meat whatsoever for the first two weeks. Within three weeks' time she had lost thirty pounds, her distressing symptoms began to disappear, and the pain in her joints was considerably reduced.

Most overweight people have unnaturally high blood pressure, and their heart action is often abnormal. If it is necessary for them to walk up a flight of stairs or move rapidly, they feel sluggish. This is because their glands and internal organs function sluggishly. When the weight is once again reduced to normal these symptoms usually disappear in a few short days.

During this 7-day miracle Oriental diet, many people who suffered from diabetes regularly checked with their doctors and found that their levels had dropped dramatically. Patients with hypoglycemia, however, are routinely advised by their doctors to use wisdom and, if necessary, some medical guidance while they are dieting. Patients who had high blood cholesterol levels when they were overweight showed dramatic reductions of this condition and returned to near-normal in a short space of time.

For centuries the world has known of the Oriental 7-day miracle diet, without realizing that it could be used to lose weight as well as to sustain a person in perfect health and with normal weight the rest of his life.

Man is by nature herbivorous and can actually subsist on a diet of vegetables, grains, fruits, and milk products. Thousands of Americans are vegetarians, eating no meat of any kind, and yet they are in splendid health, with few of the health complications we find in those who eat too much meat. Vegetarians are seldom overweight, usually have tremendous vitality, and often live to a hundred years or more.

George Bernard Shaw, the great dramatist, was a vegetarian most of his life, and lived to be nearly one hundred years old. He did his greatest work after he reached the age of sixty, and was spry, active, and had tremendous mental and physical energy. He claimed that his diet kept him in this condition.

In India, where animals (particularly cows) are considered to be sacred, little animal flesh is consumed. Instead, the sources relied upon most often for protein needs usually are a variety of nuts and seeds. Both are very capable of increasing a person's individual "energy currency," the energy created and expended between the cells themselves.

The protein and fat contained in nuts like pistachios and seeds such as sesame (both highly favored throughout India) provide tremendous fuel to the body. When other forms of food are eaten and pass through the gastrointestinal tract, there is usually some energy loss due to waste removal from the body. But the actual amount of energy lost from consumed nuts and seeds is much less than for other foods.

Here is a short list of the caloric, protein, and fat contents of some readily available nuts and seeds that you may want to incorporate into your own diet while on my efficient weight-loss plan. The information comes from John Heinerman, *Heinerman's Encyclopedia of Nuts, Berries and Seeds* (Englewood Cliffs, NJ: Prentice Hall, 1995, p. 300):

| Nuts/Seeds | Calories | Protein | Fat |
| --- | --- | --- | --- |
| Almonds | 167 | 5 grams | 15 grams |
| Cashews | 163 | 4 grams | 13 grams |
| Peanuts | 164 | 7 grams | 14 grams |
| Pecans | 187 | 2 grams | 18 grams |
| Pistachios | 162 | 6 grams | 14 grams |
| Walnuts | 182 | 4 grams | 18 grams |

■ ■ ■

## VALUABLE SOURCES OF PROTEINS

The 7-day Oriental miracle diet for losing weight does not advocate eliminating meat from the diet entirely, however. In our Western world we seem to require the important amino acids and other elements furnished by meat products. But those who are vegetarians and do not wish to eat red-blooded meats may live a long and healthy life by substituting other proteins such as grains, nuts, soybeans, milk products, and rice. Those who are vegetarians, who do not have a weight problem, may want to follow our maintenance diet, and they can be assured of having a balanced, nutritious diet that will give them health, energy, and vigor the rest of their lives.

### One Woman Lost Fifteen Pounds in Two Weeks on This Diet

On this Oriental 7-day miracle diet you may expect to lose from 7 to 15 pounds a week, depending on how rigidly you follow the diet. In the first week the average person loses about 10 pounds. Mrs. Jenny T. was 145 pounds when she began this reducing plan. She set her goal at 130 pounds, which she thought was her ideal weight, being what she weighed when she had married. She had accumulated the extra 15 pounds over a period of five years, and no amount of effort seemed to get rid of them.

Mrs. T. began the 7-day miracle diet after the two-day fasting period, which I advocate before beginning the diet. In that two-day period she did lose four pounds, but I explained to her that this was the excess salt and water held in her body tissues. Many people will lose much of this excess water in this diet in the first week, which accounts for some of the weight loss. But those who are more than 20 or 30 pounds overweight must stay on the diet a while longer than the seven days so they can lose the excess weight without endangering their health.

Then Mrs. T. began the actual Oriental diet. Within one week she had lost 7 more pounds without effort and without hunger pangs! Because she wanted to lose another four pounds she extended the Oriental diet one more week and easily lost the extra 4 pounds. Then she went on the normal maintenance diet, which she maintains to this day. She has reported to me that she has never gained back the lost pounds and that she never felt so good or had as much energy as she now has. In addition, her clothes now fit her perfectly, and she says even her romantic life has been vastly improved, and her husband finds her attractive once again.

Now that you understand the basic principles of diet and health, you are ready to embark upon the Oriental health miracle that can help you shed unwanted pounds while you retain your vital good health and still enjoy the good things life has to offer.

The following chart shows the fat content of selected foods.

## FAT CONTENT OF SELECTED ITEMS

| | |
|---|---|
| Bean curd, 4 ounces | 5 grams |
| Boiled potatoes, 1/2 cup | 0 grams |
| Butter, 1 tsp | 5 grams |
| Buttered popcorn, 3 cups | 6 grams |
| Candy apple | 0 grams |
| Caramel apple | 6 grams |
| Cheese sauce, 2 Tablespoons | 2 grams |
| Chocolate cake, 1 slice | 10 grams |
| Chocolate cream pie, 1 slice | 15 grams |
| Coleslaw, 1/2 cup | 7 grams |
| Cotton candy, one bag | 0 grams |
| Crackers, butter-type, 6 | 6 grams |
| Egg roll, one | 5+ grams |
| French fries, 10 | 15 grams |
| Fresh fruit | 0 grams |
| Fried noodles, 1 cup | 11 grams |
| Frozen fruit bar | 0 grams |
| Fruit salad | 0 grams |
| Green salad, no dressing | 0 grams |
| Ice cream, 1/2 cup | 12 grams |
| Italian bread, 1 chunk | 0 grams |
| Lentil soup, 1 cup | 3 grams |
| Macaroni and cheese, 6 ounces | 19 grams |
| Macaroni salad, 1/2 cup | 12 grams |
| Margarine, one pat | 5 grams |
| Marinara sauce, 1/2 cup | 4 grams |
| Mayonnaise-based dressing, regular, 1 T | 6 grams |
| Mayonnaise-based dressing, reduced-calorie, 1 T | 2 grams |
| Melba toast, saltine crackers (4) | trace |
| Minestrone soup, 1 cup | 3 grams |

## FAT CONTENT OF SELECTED ITEMS
*(cont'd)*

| | |
|---|---|
| Mozzarella cheese, 1 oz. | 8 grams |
| Oil-based salad dressing, regular, 1 T. | 9 grams |
| Oil-based dressing, reduced-calorie, 1 T | 3 grams |
| Olive oil, 1 tsp. | 5 grams |
| Olives, 10 small or 5 large | 5 grams |
| Parmezan cheese, 2 T. | 3 grams |
| Pasta salad, $^1/_2$ cup | 5+ grams |
| Peanuts, $^1/_4$ cup | 18 grams |
| Plain fruits and vegetables (such as carrots, green peppers, mushrooms, beets, grapes). | 0 grams |
| Plain pasta, 1 cup | 1 gram |
| Potato chips, 1 ounce (about 15 - 20 chips). | 10 grams |
| Ricotta cheese, 2 T. | 3 grams |
| Shredded cheddar cheese, $^1/_4$ cup or 4 T | 9 grams |
| Soft noodles (lo mein) 1 cup | 2 grams |
| Steamed rice $^1/_2$ cup. | 0 grams |
| Steamed vegetables, plain | 0 grams |
| Sunflower seeds, 1 T. | 5 grams |
| Three-bean salad, $^1/_2$ cup. | 3+ grams |
| Unbuttered popcorn, 3 cups | 0 grams |
| Vegetables, (broccoli, snow peas, water chestnuts, carrots, bok choy) | 0 grams |

# CHAPTER 2

# TAKING THE FIRST STEPS TO LOSE FROM TEN TO TWENTY POUNDS WITHOUT EFFORT

T■ ■ ■

he basic foundation of the Oriental 7-day miracle diet is one of natural foods, made up mainly of vegetables, fruits, grains, and brown rice, with the addition of fish, fowl, or other protein meats. Although rice is thought of as a carbohydrate food, the natural brown rice, which has not been polished, contains many nutrients, including protein, that are valuable as food and are not converted into fat.

This diet, which includes brown rice, must not be confused with other diets that concentrate only on rice. It is true that rice, when used as an adjunct in a reducing diet, gives that full feeling which helps one resist the tendency to overeat. However, rice alone does not provide balanced nutrition. This is why I have added other foods to our quick-reducing system.

For centuries two-thirds of the world's population has lived on a predominantly rice diet. Rice and vegetables, with some meat, fish, milk products, and eggs, have been used as the sustaining diet of millions of people in the Far East. You seldom see a fat person in the Far Eastern countries.

I observed in my travels throughout the Far East and India that the rural people who did not have access to the processed and refined or canned foods of the cities subsisted entirely on the simple products they were able to raise—mainly rice, vegetables, fruits, and grains in their natural state.

I checked with medical authorities and hospital records in these countries and discovered a strange thing: Despite the fact that these people knew little about hygienic laws, which accounted for many deaths among children, they often lived to be one hundred or more years of age.

The records showed that these people, who lived solely on the natural foods they grew, such as grains and vegetables, had little or no cardiac disease, and high blood pressure was practically unknown. These is less incidence of cancer, arthritis, sugar diabetes, and other diseases associated with being overweight among these country people.

■ ■ ■

## THE VITAL IMPORTANCE OF RICE IN WEIGHT REDUCTION

Dr. Jeffrey S. Bland, a nutritional authority who is well recognized in the American health food industry, has characterized rice as "the wonder food" of all time. In an article on this subject in the November 1995 issue of *Let's Live* magazine (pp. 26–27) he listed some of his reasons for making this statement. For one, a large number of Americans and their children are hypersensitive to the gluten in grains such as wheat, corn, oats, and barley. They frequently experience diarrhea, bloating, gas, and stomach pains as a result of consuming such foods.

But rice is one of the very few grains that doesn't bother them. This is because it lacks gluten, the hypersensitizing protein that produces such allergic reactions in people with a genetic sensitivity to it. Rice can even help to promote better digestion, because its carbohydrates are so "user-friendly" to the digestive tract.

In addition, Dr. Bland cited evidence from McGill University– Montreal Children's Hospital in eastern Canada to show that rice contains substances that help to normalize intestinal functions. Anyone suffering from *any* type of gastrointestinal discomfort should give serious consideration to rice, he concludes.

According to an article written by Allen Simon in the May/June 1982 issue of *The Saturday Evening Post* (p. 102), rice is "the almost perfect health food" for those intending to diet, but not wanting to give up too many of the things they enjoy eating. He noted that rice "is a natural for what nutritionists call 'protein sparing.' This means simply that, by eating rice with your meal, you can safely cut down on your meat portion." He goes on to say that the rice will furnish a person's energy needs while at the same time the small amount of protein in the meat "can be used for what it does best," namely to repair cells. "The result," he adds, "is a better balanced meal, with less fat and cholesterol."

Moreover, *rice isn't fattening* like many other energy-producing foods are. Just look at the hundreds of millions of people throughout the Orient and other Third World countries who consume large helpings of rice at every meal. Very few of them ever show signs of obesity, and those of the modern generation who do are usually guilty of subsisting on many "fast foods" from America. When Dr. Earl Mindell (author of the bestseller *The Vitamin Bible*) and I went to Japan with some other scientists a few years ago, we were amazed to see just how slender most Japanese men and women were who spanned the ages of thirty to fifty-five. As long as they stayed with their traditional diet of rice, they didn't gain any extra weight. But the moment they began indulging themselves in McDonalds hamburgers, Kentucky Fried Chicken, Taco Bell bean burritos, or Ben & Jerry's ice cream, their weight began to increase.

The Chinese and the Japanese, more than any other ethnic groups in the Orient, virtually worship this ancient grain. In 500 B.C. Confucius considered rice to be the necessary and appropriate food for the virtuous and graceful life. That's probably why so many Chinese eat upward of 515 pounds of rice per person every year! Americans, on the other hand, consume an average of only 17 pounds per year. In Japan, *okome*—"honorable rice"—is anything but a commodity. In the Shinto religion, sake, rice cakes, and other rice products are the most sacred offerings. To politicians, rice is a symbol of independence to a nation that must import much of its meat, fish, and fruit. During our two-week stay in Japan, I witnessed several taste testers checking *gohan*, or steamed rice, in restaurants for the proper stickiness. And I had a chance to visit several stores called *komeya* that sold nothing but rice. Like wine shops, they offer many varieties, identified by strain and home regions.

A decade before my trip to Japan, I had a chance to tour mainland China with members of the American Medical Students' Association. Everywhere our group of twenty-nine medical students and four faculty advisors (myself included) went we were offered rice, rice, and more rice. There was rice for breakfast, rice for lunch, rice for dinner, and rice to snack on. No wonder the Chinese people seemed so healthy and *so lean*. Chinese doctors with whom we spoke through the assistance of translators at the Shanghai Second Medical College informed us that rice had helped to keep heart disease, hypertension, diabetes, and obesity to a minimum in their country in comparison with Europe and North America. We were convinced that rice was, indeed, "a serious food miracle for good health management" (as one doctor put it).

One of the really important things about rice that my visits to China, Japan, and a number of other Oriental counties over the years has taught me is the *proper* way in which it is prepared. The makeup of the starch in the rice kernel determines the cooking quality. Actually, the important factor is really the percentage of the principal starch component called amylose. If that percentage is low, say 10 to 18 percent, the rice tends to be soft and somewhat sticky; the way the Japanese, Koreans, Taiwanese, and Chinese like it. On the other hand, if it's high, say 25 to 30 percent, the rice will be hard and fluffy, which suits the taste buds of Indians, Pakistanis, and Sri Lankans just fine. The preference of Southeast Asians—Indonesians, Thais, Malaysians—is somewhere in between, as is that of Americans and Europeans. Laotians prefer their rice with an extra-low amylose content, about 2 percent, or very sticky, glutinous, gluey, *but* with every kernel distinct.

So if you're served a clump of mushy, shapeless rice, don't blame the amylose; blame the chef instead. That rice was cooked with too much water, or simply too long—and when that occurs, it will come out mushy every time, no matter what its starch composition may be.

Few foods are as intimidating to cook as this grain seems to be. The proliferation of "fool-proof" precooked varieties is testimony enough to that. But those products can be bland and rubbery. You can pass them up and produce first-rate long-cooking rice by following a few simple suggestions. This information was gleaned first-hand from informants in Bali, Myanmar, Thailand, Laos, Vietnam, China, Korea, Japan, and Taiwan, who cook rice several times every day for their meals.

By following these few general rules, from the experts in the Orient who know rice well, you won't end up with something that's too mushy or too dry, but just right. And it will provide you with a wonderful food alternative and nifty side dish for many meals, keeping you slim and trim.

*Rule #1:* Use $1^3/_4$ cups (not the commonly suggested 2) of very hot or boiling water per cup of uncooked rice. Most top-rated products—those least sticky, starchy, and mushy—recommend hot-water starts. A cup of raw rice will yield about 4 cups of cooked rice. A cup of uncooked instant rice will yield 2 cups.

*Rule #2: Never* permit rice to go into a full, rolling boil, so my Oriental informants told me. They all warned that doing so would rupture the grains and produce a starchy mass.

*Rule #3:* My friends along the Pacific Rim said that rice is best cooked at a very low simmer. Higher heat will cause the grains to stick to the pot.

*Rule #4:* Let the finished product absorb residual moisture by keeping it tightly covered and off the heat for 5 minutes. If it's still too damp, fluff it with a fork, return the lid, and leave the pot over very low heat for another couple of minutes.

As for cooking time and heat settings, each of my informants had a different set of specifications for this. But as you get the hang of it, you'll discover the time and temperature that's best for the type of rice you're using and the area of the country you live in.

■ ■ ■

## RICE CREATIONS THAT WILL KEEP YOU HEALTHY, HAPPY, AND HEARTY WITHOUT EVER GAINING A SINGLE POUND

I'm so excited about rice and what it has done for thousands of people who've tried my Oriental 7-day quick weight-off diet for themselves and lost pounds in just a matter of a week, that I just have to share some great recipes with you right now. Ordinarily, I'd wait until later in the book to do this, where you'll find many other wonderful recipes. But this seemed as appropriate as any place to introduce you to some fantastic dishes that are going to fill you up, *but not out!*

First, let's briefly examine the types of rice available in most markets at present. There's long-grain rice that's four to five times as long as it is wide. Its grains stay separate when cooked and work well in curries or pilafs. Long-grain white rice is what's left after the hull, bran and germ of the grain are removed. The grains are long, thin, and usually opaque. The flavor is mild, and the texture is fluffy, with a touch of stickiness.

Next comes brown rice, which is hulled, but still contains the germ and bran. It contains twice as much fiber, five times as much vitamin E content and three times as much magnesium as white rice. Long-grain brown rice is fluffy, with a sometimes nutty flavor; short-grain brown rice has a similar flavor, but its texture is denser and chewier.

Now we come to basmati rice from India or Pakistan; this is very white and, when cooked, very long. Its flavor is delicate; its aroma is nutty during cooking. Basmati means "queen of fragrance," and this aromatic rice is eaten on special occasions in India. There's also American basmati rice, grown mostly in Texas, which is light, fluffy, and aromatic, with a stronger flavor than its Indian or Pakistani counterparts.

Medium-grain rice tends to be plumper and more tender than the long-grain rices. Most are grown in Italy and Spain—regions located farther away from the equator. Spanish rice, grown in Valencia, is a medium-grain rice that suits paella, a dish of rice and seafood. Arborio is a medium-grain, shiny rice from Italy. It develops a sticky, creamy texture when cooked.

Short-grain rice is almost round. It's softer than long- or medium-grain rice and works well for sushi or rice pudding. Glutinous rice is quite sticky, and due to its sweet flavor, is most often used in making desserts. Finally, converted rice has been steam-treated before milling, pushing nutrients from the bran into the grain. Uncle Ben's Converted Rice is probably the best known brand of this type of rice.

A word or two ought to be said about wild rice, which isn't rice at all, nor is it consumed anywhere in Asia. It's actually the seed of a native North American grass and has been a favorite of Great Lakes Indian tribes for many centuries. Still, it is classified as a grain, and for all intents and purposes, wild rice is cooked and treated just like all other rice varieties, except that it requires more water and a longer cooking time. Packages will give you full instructions, but generally the ratio is one part wild rice to three parts liquid. Cooking times can range from thirty-five minutes to one hour. When it comes to flavor and texture, wild rice is like a dark, distant, mysterious cousin of the white rice that Orientals favor. It has an inherently different flavor profile—a chewy texture and a pleasing, earthy aroma. The most preferred wild rice is that harvested from Minnesota or another Great Lakes state, even though California remains the major producer of this grain at present. Here's a little culinary tidbit I'm passing along to you, in the event that you can afford this very expensive rice: try pairing wild rice with wild mushrooms or sweet dried fruits such as prunes, apricots, dates, or raisins. Trust me on this one, because you're in for the gourmet treat of your life!

I'm indebted to Shizuo Tsuji for some of the following rice dishes. Some twenty years ago he was in charge of the École Technique Hôtelière Tsuji in Osaka, that largest school for professional chefs in Japan. To this day, I still remember his favorite expression, uttered with the dignity that one might expect from such a distinguished food connoisseur: "Rice is a very beautiful food. It is beautiful when it grows, beautiful when harvested, and beautiful when threshed. But, most of all, it is at its greatest beauty when cooked by a practiced hand, so pure and snow white and sweetly fragrant."

### TAI MESHI
*(Sea Bass and Rice)*

1 whole sea bass, about 8 inches in length

$2^1/_2$ cups short-grain rice, washed

$3^1/_3$ cups *dashi* (chicken broth)

1 Tbsp. dried, powdered *hijiki* (a popular brown algae that is sold in Japanese and Korean markets in major cities)

2 Tbsp. dark or light soy sauce

5 drops of *mirin* (sweet cooking sake)

Scale and gut the fish, but keep head and tail intact. Skewer the fish as follows: Using two long metal skewers, begin skewering from the tail forward, as well as from beneath the eye backward. Then prick the skin a few times with a needle to prevent it from blistering and shrinking. Lightly season the tail and fins with some ground hijiki. Grill over a medium-hot charcoal fire or broil in a preheated oven. Grill on both sides, turning once, until almost done, about 8 minutes on each side, depending on the level of the heat and thickness of the fish.

Next, put the washed rice into a 10-inch earthenware casserole (or any other kind of casserole that can take direct flame and has a snug-fitting lid). Add the *dashi*, the rest of the *hijiki*, the soy sauce, and *mirin*, and stir. Place the grilled fish in the center (the stock will cover about half of it).

Put the lid on and cook until the liquid comes to a vigorous boil; the lid might bounce from the pressure of the steam. Turn off the heat and leave the casserole dish standing for 15 minutes undisturbed. Flake the fish with a dinner fork to remove the bones. Mix it with the rice. Serves about 4.

## KURI GOHAN
*(Chestnut Rice)*

15 large, fresh chestnuts (in season in late September or early October)

$1/2$ tsp. salt

4 cups water

$31/3$ cups short-grain rice, washed

Carefully shell the chestnuts and remove the thin inner skin. You need a very sharp paring knife for this. Cut them into quarters. Try not to let them crumble into bits—these will disintegrate when cooked later on. Rinse pared, cut-up chestnuts in cold water to remove their starch, then drain.

Use an earthenware casserole, a heavy pot with a tight-fitting lid, or an electric or gas rice cooker. If you don't already have one on hand, visit a Japanese or Korean market and inquire about where to buy one of these.

Dissolve the salt in the water, then pour over the rice in the cooking vessel. Add the chestnuts, cover, and cook in the same manner as described for Tai Meshi. Let stand, covered, 15 minutes before serving. Serve hot in individual bowls. Serves about 4.

## OYAKO DONBURI
*(Chicken-'n-Egg on Rice)*

6–8 cups hot, cooked rice

4–5 eggs

$1/4$ lb. chicken

4 green onions

*Sauce:*

$21/2$ cups *dashi* (chicken stock)

6 Tbsp. dark and 3 Tbsp. light soy sauce

3 Tbsp. honey

Prepare the plain white rice according to instructions on the package or previously given in this chapter.

Mix but don't beat the eggs with a fork and set aside.

Cut the boned chicken (without skin) into $1/4$ inch pieces. The chicken should be raw, but if your purpose for making this dish is to use leftovers, cooked chicken is fine, as is thin-sliced raw or cooked pork or beef. The flavor is best if you start with raw meat, however.

Wash and clean the onions. Cut them diagonally into 1-inch lengths.

Combine the ingredients for the sauce in a medium-sized saucepan. Bring the contents to a gentle boil over medium heat. Add the chicken and simmer, uncovered, for 5 minutes. Then add the onion and simmer a minute longer. Correct the seasoning, if necessary.

Stir the eggs again and gently pour them in a steady stream around the chicken in the simmering sauce. Let the egg spread naturally. *Do not stir.* Keep the heat at medium until the egg starts to bubble at the edges. At this point, stir once. The egg will have almost set but still be a little runny. Keep in mind that the high temperature of the rice over which the egg will be placed will do the final cooking. Be careful, however, that you don't let the egg cook hard.

Put portions of hot rice, $1^1/_2$ to 2 cups, into individual soup bowls. With a large spoon, scoop a portion of the egg topping and sauce and place on the rice. The sauce will seep down into the rice, but the dish will not be soupy. Serves 4.

### OISHII KOME KYABETSU
*(Cole Slaw with Rice)*

2 cups brown rice, cooked

$1/_2$ small red cabbage, shredded to make about 3 cups

2 carrots, finely julienned

1 small red onion, thinly sliced

1 medium bulb fennel, halved lengthwise and thinly sliced
    (about 2 cups)

1 tsp. each caraway seed and pepper

$^1/_4$ cup each balsamic vinegar and olive oil

2 Tbsp. each dijon mustard and olive oil

In a large bowl, toss all ingredients together well and let stand for 35 minutes before serving. Makes approximately 8 cups.

■ ■ ■

## ADDING MEATS FOR PROTEIN NEEDS

In my Oriental 7-day diet, I recognize the need for meat proteins. However, I advocate the splendid protein to be found in fish. In fact the Japanese diet consisting mostly of fish, rice, and vegetables is probably one of the most nourishing of all, for fish have been found to be a better form of protein than that of the red-blooded meats!

These fine foods, which are nourishing and which are included in my 7-day reducing diet, not only cause you to lose weight when eaten as directed, but when you have reached your desired normal weight, furnish you body with all the necessary vitamins, minerals, and other elements you need in a normal diet. They will also keep you from becoming overweight again. The Japanese are noted for their slender, wiry figures; seldom do you see an overweight Japanese person.

Have you had the experience of eating in a Chinese or Japanese restaurant? After eating several courses consisting of rice, vegetables, soup, and lean meat, you felt stuffed and thought you would not want to eat again for days. Then a few hours later you experienced hunger once more.

The explanation is simple: you actually receive very little fat-producing food in such an Oriental diet, but you do receive plenty of bulk. The egg drop soup has little fat content; the vegetables are mostly boiled; the meat is usually lean and broiled; then when you add three or four cups of tea to the meal, you experience that stuffed feeling that makes you think you have had a hearty feast. This is one of the reasons for the popularity of Chinese and Japanese restaurants in this country.

My Oriental 7-day miracle diet is based on this basic Oriental diet, which extends throughout the Orient, including China, Japan, India, Tibet, Indonesia, Vietnam, and Cambodia, and also other countries in the Near East and Far East that use rice as their staple diet.

However, to this diet I have added another important ingredient, which helps you lose weight quickly and without hunger: it is a method of fixing the numerous vegetables that give bulk without giving weight, in a simple manner that requires no special cooking and that furnishes you with the bulk that takes away hunger pangs.

■ ■ ■

## EAT AS MUCH AS YOU WISH AND LOSE WEIGHT

I promised you that you can, with this miracle diet, *eat as much as you wish and still lose weight.* Also, that you need never be hungry while on this reducing diet. Now let me explain this more fully before you start on the actual reducing plan.

On this diet, the nonfattening vegetables I shall give you require more calories to digest than they give your body in caloric value. This is one of the secrets of the effectiveness of my 7-day quick weight-loss diet.

When a farmer wants to fatten a pig what does he do? He gives the pig plenty of corn and other fat-producing foods and shuts it up in a small space so it cannot get much exercise, and in a few weeks' time it will be as fat as a—pig!

In dieting to lose weight, you must eat these weight-reducing vegetables each day as a supplement to the other foods given in the reducing list. The easiest and quickest way to utilize these weight-reducing vegetables is to put them into a soup and then eat all the soup you want, as many times a day as you feel hungry. This is why I said that you may eat as much as up to five or six pounds of food a day and eat as often as you feel hungry of these weight-reducing vegetables without putting on an ounce! The vegetables in the list I give below for making the reducing soup take more calories to digest than they give to the body! *The more of these vegetables you eat the more you lose!*

### How to Prepare the Reducing Soup

Prepare the following vegetables by cleaning them and cutting them up into medium-sized pieces.

1 head of cabbage

6 large onions

A big bunch of celery

A big green pepper

A can of whole tomatoes

After you have cut up these vegetables, place them in a large pot, cover them over with water, and let the water come to a full boil. After it has boiled about 10 minutes lower the fire and let the reducing soup simmer for a full $2^1/_2$ to 3 hours, or until the vegetables are soft. Do not worry that you will be cooking all the nutrients out of the vegetables! This soup is not intended to nourish you! *In fact, if you ate nothing but this soup you would soon starve to death!* It will give no nourishment and no fat to the body whatsoever, which is why it is used, but it will give you the comfortable feeling of being full, and you can eat it as often as you wish when you feel hungry, with the other basic reducing foods I shall give you in a few moments. When you eat a bowl of this reducing soup you may sprinkle it with Parmesan cheese to make it more palatable. You can also add a small container of onion soup mix, which can be found in your grocery store, just to give it more flavor. This should be done while the big pot of soup is cooking. The reason I suggest preparing a big pot of this reducing soup is that it is easy to prepare and to keep for days in your refrigerator, saving you the bother of making it every day.

To give you full nutritional value on this reducing diet, I shall add other basic foods that will give your body the nourishment you require without adding to your body weight.

This reducing soup is to be eaten between meals. You may eat your regular meals three times a day, and in addition, three or four bowls of the reducing soup, as often as you wish and you will actually lose weight quickly!

The wonderful thing about using this reducing soup is that it will fill you up so much that you will have no feeling or appetite for the carbohydrates and other fat-producing foods. All foods produce fats when they are eaten in large quantities—even lean meats. Many people believe that eating lean meat and vegetables alone, all they want, will cause them to lose weight. But if they eat more than 900 calories each day they will not lose weight. During this critical seven-day period the actual food intake is kept to less than 1,000 calories a day. However, you do not need to count calories, as this will be automatic in the quantities suggested in this reducing diet. Later, however, I shall have something to say about calories and their importance in adjusting to your regular maintenance diet, after you have shed the unwanted pounds.

■ ■ ■

## FASTING REGIME TO BEGIN LOSING WEIGHT IMMEDIATELY

To begin losing weight immediately and to convert the foods you eat into solid protein without fat, you should begin your diet regime with the system used in most of the Far Eastern countries: this is to fast and drink only liquids and fruit or vegetable juices. This system of purification of the body is essential before starting to reduce. It will help you rid the body of all accumulated wastes and poisons. It will also help you remove several pounds of excess liquids that may lodge in the body cells, held there by salt that you have eaten for years. If this fasting regime is not followed, the body is not prepared to absorb the new elements introduced into it through the diet, and many of the body's previous inflammations and congestions are apt to remain.

I have observed in many of the religious orders of the Far East that the monks observe regular periods of fasting for as long as two or three weeks at a time, with only a daily intake of water, and fruit and vegetable juices. Many of these monks live to be more than a hundred years of age and have perfect health, with slender bodies and youthful appearance. Fasting was one of Gandhi's secrets for energy, health, and long life.

■ ■ ■

## SHORT JUICE FASTS: AN EASY, PAINLESS WAY OF DETOXIFICATION AND LOSING WEIGHT

Mahatma Gandhi was also a vegetarian most of his life, and when he was assassinated, even though he was in his early seventies, the doctors said that his body was like that of a man in his thirties. Gandhi used certain principles of our Oriental diet, and was famous for his long fasts, during which he ate no solid foods, subsisting only on diluted orange juice and water.

The practice of fasting is as old as civilization itself. In ancient times, fasting was done for one of two reasons: either involuntarily during periods of food scarcity; or for religious purposes. In those instances, spiritual communication of some sort was usually desired with the god or gods being worshipped.

A minister once said in connection with fasting and prayer: "Fasting and prayer go together. Fasting is when you give up something important to the flesh (namely, food) in order to spend that time with God. But those who fast and maintain their regular activities during a fast are not fasting but are only *dieting*." This section of this book covers fasting in relation to weight loss, of course. But the good pastor's observations of prayer in connection with fasting are worth considering, especially in light of what we now know about the connection between the mind and the body. Exploring the religious dimension while you are on my Oriental 7-day diet isn't going to hurt you one bit; in fact, it may do wonders for your soul, besides giving you the type of slender figure you're after.

Many religions the world over routinely prescribe some type of fasting, teaching that it is good not only for the body but also for the soul of the individual. Once a month members of the Church of Jesus Christ of Latter-Day Saints set aside the consumption of two meals and give the dollar equivalent thereof to their church leaders to help the poor. Pope John Paul II once said that "contemporary people must fast, that is, abstain not only from food and beverages but from many other means of consumptions, stimulation, and satisfaction of the senses." Members of the Hare Krishna sect engage in brief fasts several times a month. For example, September third is Annada Ekadasi, or fasting from grains and beans; September fourteenth is fasting until noon, followed by feasting on Sri Radhastami's Day; and September twenty-second is considered to be "the third month of Caturmasya," which begins the fasting from milk.

The length of the fast may vary, depending on who's doing it and his or her religious beliefs. According to the sacred book of the ancient Maya, called the *Popol Vuh,* "The Quiche lords fasted for 180 days, burned offerings, and then fasted 260 days more (eating dried fruits—mammee, soursop, and custard apples). Sometimes they [even] fasted for 340 days. [During this time] they made [religious] vows, abstained from sexual relations, and remained in [their] temples." (This is according to information furnished by anthropologist Sandra L. Orellana in her book *The Tzutujil Mayas: Continuity and Change, 1250-1630* (Norman: University of Oklahoma Press, 1984; p. 101.) The late black human rights activist and actor Dick Gregory claimed that in his lifetime, "I've fasted over 150 times; I've addressed everything from world hunger to violence." Periodic fasting helped him to shed more than two hundred pounds of ugly fat (he once weighed close to four hundred pounds when he was about thirty-five years of age, believe it or not!).

Lengthy fasts, though, are definitely hazardous to the health of the average person. And more so to those suffering from blood sugar problems like diabetes or hypoglycemia, where continued nourishment is of primary importance for maintenance of general health. Through trial and error, however, Gregory managed to bring a sense of balance to his method of fasting—something, by the way, that he didn't advocate that everybody do.

He told us once in an interview: "The best way to lose weight is to drink a minimum of eight glasses of water, eat fruit for breakfast, fruit for lunch, and one meal in the evening consisting of rice. I always recommend that a good vitamin-and-mineral supplement be taken when doing this. The important thing here is never to go below 800 calories a day. When we go below this line, the brain panics and sends a message to the body that there's a famine, because the brain doesn't know you're fat. Then your weight loss stops, and your body holds the fat now to protect your life. But, if you keep it at 1,000 calories, and basically eat apples, bananas, carrots, celery, potatoes, and things like that there's enough alkalinity and fiber there to release the natural sugar in these things more gradually through the body over a longer period of time, so that your sugar level doesn't decrease. That's what makes people get so hungry in the first place, when their sugar levels drop like crazy. But doing it my way prevents that from happening."

People who want to start my Oriental 7-day quick weight-off diet and know about the fasting aspect of it often ask me, "Does my stomach really shrink when I don't eat for a while?" I end up telling them that, in a sense, it does. I explain that the stomach does contract when it's empty, and that's one of the reasons it takes so little food to fill you up after you go a day or so without eating. But there's a biochemical reason for the phenomenon as well.

People should thing of their stomachs as elastic sacks. Go ahead and enjoy a good-sized serving of fettucini Alfredo, a glass of wine or beer, and a piece of fruit—about a quart and a half of food, counting the digestive juices—and your sack will fill just to the comfort point.

That pressure will send your brain a subtle signal to turn down your appetite, although you can keep eating, I suppose, if you have a problem with gluttony. The muscles in the walls of your stomach can easily stretch, even to an astonishing degree. Your stomach can readily accommodate more than a gallon of food and liquid, though a meal that size will leave you feeling uncomfortably full.

A mere two hours later, your stomach should be fairly empty. But if you fast for twenty-four hours or so, your stomach will collapse on itself like a wrinkled balloon. Now, just a couple of bites of pasta can leave you feeling satiated, as those morsels make room for themselves by pushing at the stomach's lining.

The late health guru Paavo Airola advocated no more than a three-day period of fasting for those without medical problems who were serious about losing weight. He taught his patients a great deal about whole foods and an improved diet, which prepared their bodies for the trauma of weight loss. Often people just start dieting without any thought about the trauma it can cause the system. That's why it's a good idea to "prep" the body first by *slowly* phasing in dieting. Dr. Airola placed his subjects on a program of drinking lemon juice and water one day a week. He usually chose the weekend for this.

Part of his regimen was to drink lemon juice (one lemon squeezed into thirty-two ounces of distilled water, plus a touch of honey if desired) alternately with one quart of plain, distilled water. The purpose of this combination was to cleanse the body. He noted that the lemon has a powerful cleansing action on the system, especially for those in a highly toxic state.

Because most of his patients had to drink the lemon juice mixture every hour on the hour and the distilled water every hour on the half hour, they hardly had any time to think about being hungry. A number of those who had been on his "phase-in dieting" (as he called it) confided to me some years later than they were often too busy either using the bathroom or napping to have much on an appetite for anything.

By the end of their twenty-four-hour juice fasts, they reported feeling refreshed and rested, with very few side effects such as nausea, headaches, or stomach discomfort. (The only "negative" side effect, if it can be called that, was their constant use of the bathroom. But since this really wasn't a painful effect, and it indicated that the body was cleansing itself, it was viewed more as positive but sometimes inconvenient.) No one that I interviewed who had been on Dr. Airola's short fast ever complained of feeling ill. By the time they were ready to start with his three-day juice fasting, their bodies had already become somewhat detoxified and, essentially, *prepared* for the dieting experience itself.

Dr. Airola always insisted that his patients do their fasting on a Friday–Saturday–Sunday weekend, when there would be no real output of physical energy. He divided the juices into two categories: fruit juices were the *cleansers* of the system, while vegetable juices were the *regenerators*. He had his patients alternate between the two, which is what I've advocated in my own diet program here. People have reported experiencing more energy and with it an accompanying feeling of lightness as well. As the late health pioneer Paul Bragg was fond of saying, even well into his nineties: "Fasting renovates, revives and purifies each and every one of the millions of cells that make up the human body."

Well, I can assure you that you will notice the benefits of a short juice fast very quickly. You will feel like eating less even, in some cases developing a mild aversion to those junk foods you once craved. But you will have more bounce in your step and feel an exhilaration that is nearly indescribable.

■ ■ ■

## NOW YOU ARE READY TO BEGIN YOUR WEIGHT-REDUCING PROGRAM

When you have concluded your fasting period you are ready to embark upon your regular 7-day reducing regimen.

First, I would suggest that you try to rid your diet of regular table salt, which is sodium chloride, and use some of the salt substitutes on the market. Salt has the peculiar faculty of holding water in the body tissues, which often accounts for from five to ten pounds of excessive weight! More and more nutritionists and doctors are advising against the use of table salt, stressing how it affects blood pressure and is a prime suspect in many cases of arthritis and other diseases. If there is any doubt in your case, do not hesitate to consult your doctor to see if your condition requires special salt restrictions.

The body needs sodium, it is true, but not sodium chloride, which is labeled as a poison in drug stores! Sodium is easily obtainable in many of the vegetables we shall use in our reducing diet, including summer squash or zucchini, and green string beans, as well as celery and other green vegetables.

To begin your reducing diet you must eat certain reducing vegetables and avoid the starchy vegetables, which add weight to your body.

■ ■ ■

## THE BASIC ORIENTAL WEIGHT-REDUCING DIET

The basic element in this 7-day Oriental reducing diet, as I have stated before, is rice, especially brown rice. The vegetables are eaten in your soup, and therefore I shall not include them in planning your three meals a day for the seven-day period you want to lose weight.

However, later I shall give you many variations to this rice diet, and many vegetables for the sustaining diet, which are nourishing and tasty, cooked as the Orientals cook them, and these will give you variety in menu planning without adding fat to your body.

For Breakfast: Start your day with a good solid breakfast. This is one of the most important meals of the day. Many people skimp on breakfast and think they are losing weight; actually, avoiding a hearty breakfast accounts for many cases of fatigue and headache and makes people turn quarrelsome and highly nervous. The reason for this is that during the long period of time when you sleep, the body is without food which tends to lower the blood sugar level. Upon rising in the morning, after taking a small glass of orange or grapefruit juice, half an hour before your breakfast, you will be much more receptive to a solid breakfast.

Then eat two boiled, poached, or fried eggs. Be sure the eggs are fried without grease. Coated pans are excellent for greaseless cooking. Then have one piece of whole-wheat toast with butter, a half spoonful of any kind of jelly or marmalade, and all the coffee you want, if you drink it black and without sugar. However, you may use cream, but with artificial sweetener. The sugar is more harmful than the cream, for your body needs some fat each day, even when you are reducing. You may take this fat as cream in your coffee or tea, or as butter on your toast.

Brown rice is not suggested for the morning meal as it is apt to make you feel too full so early in the morning, but it can be used later in the day, either for lunch or for dinner.

If you have breakfast around 7 A.M. you will begin to feel hungry again within a period of three or four hours. Then you can eat a big bowl of the vegetable reducing soup, sprinkled with Parmesan cheese for flavoring. This soup in itself tastes delicious, for the onions give it flavor. Eat as much as you wish or until your hunger pangs go away.

If you go to work and cannot prepare this at home for midmorning to relieve hunger, you can take a bowl of the vegetable soup in a thermos jug and eat it at your place of business before your regular lunch.

It was found by scientists investigating the food habits of people all over the world that the country people in Bulgaria, Romania, Yugoslavia, Russia, and the other countries in the area often ate nothing all day but vegetable soup, brown bread, milk products and cheese, yogurt, and eggs—with very little meat—and they found that many of these people lived as long as 125 to 135 years. They were slender, youthful appearing, and often worked in the fields all day up to an advanced age!

### The Importance of Brown Rice

In addition to the reducing soup you are now ready to add the brown rice to your diet. This will be a staple part of your diet while losing weight. Many people think of rice as being starchy, forgetting that the natural brown rice, when it is not ruined by refining and polishing, has valuable proteins and other elements that make it an ideal food.

You may eat a helping of brown rice, a cupful at least, with butter on it, at lunch or dinner. This basic staple food will give you a feeling of fullness and help keep you from growing hungry. Sometimes for lunch or dinner you can eat a big bowlful of brown rice with a poached egg on it and a little melted butter. It will give you tremendous energy and stamina without that feeling of weakness in the knees than often comes when one is on a stringent weight-reducing diet.

Prepare a large bowl of brown rice by cooking it with a little salt substitute, for about forty-five minutes. If you cannot get brown rice you can use white rice, although it is not as valuable as a food staple. When the rice is cooked, put it in the refrigerator and twice a day, for lunch and for dinner, warm a small bowlful, about a cup and a half, and add a little melted butter for flavor. You can eat as much of this rice as you feel gives you a completely satisfied feeling. With the rice you can also eat a four-ounce piece of lean meat, such as veal, beef, or lamb, or a piece of chicken with the skin removed, broiled or baked. All meats should be broiled or boiled, never fried.

The diet can be varied each day by having a different form of meat. If you are a vegetarian you can eat a meat substitute made from soybeans, or you may use cottage cheese, eggs, or skim milk.

During this period of dieting eat no cake, pie, or ice cream. No desserts of any kind are permitted, except natural fruits or Jello made with natural gelatin and artificial sweetener. You may add fruits to it, but if they are canned fruits, the syrup should be washed off of them or you may use the canned dietetic fruits that contain artificial sweetener.

For desserts you may also eat stewed apples or apple sauce. You can add a little honey or use artificial sweetener. You may also eat apricots, prunes, cantaloupe, watermelon, strawberries, cherries, honeydew melon, and rhubarb. These are the only fruits permitted while on this reducing diet. All the above fruits are wonderful while reducing, for they do not add calories because they require more calories to digest than they give to the body. Other fruits are prohibited while on the weight-reducing diet.

If you feel the need for other desserts while reducing, you may eat fat-free yogurt, which you can mix with fruit. But remember, yogurt is easily digested and assimilated, so do not overindulge in such foods while dieting!

For Lunch: You are permitted a large serving of cottage cheese with fresh fruit; a salad with a nonfattening salad dressing, which I shall give later; a piece of fish or lean meat, and a piece of whole-wheat bread with a pat of butter. You may drink coffee or tea, without cream. Or you may use a nondairy cream with artificial sweetening.

You can satisfy your hunger by adding to this luncheon a bowl of the reducing soup and also a cupful of brown rice, flavored with melted butter. When you eat this type of lunch, you will have a stuffed feeling, but you will have actually eaten nothing that will add fat to your body. To avoid overeating you can take the bowl of reducing soup about an hour or so before lunch or dinner; in this way you will help kill your appetite and will not have a desire for much solid food.

For Dinner: Have a bowl of the reducing soup a short time before dinner to kill your appetite. You can then have a helping of one of the meats given above; a small salad of tomatoes, cucumbers, and lettuce; and for dessert a bowl of sugar-free Jello, or some fruit, such as applesauce or melon.

Potatoes are not permitted in this reducing diet. However, if you want to add vegetables to this diet and not eat the reducing soup with your dinner, you may have two helpings of any of these vegetables: broccoli, string beans, asparagus, zucchini, spinach, turnips, or tomatoes. This gives you a wide variety of the reducing vegetables to eat, if you prepare them without sauces or starchy fillers. They can be steamed until soft and then flavored with a little margarine, or one of the nonfattening sauces I shall give later.

■ ■ ■

## FOODS TO AVOID DURING THIS 7-DAY REDUCING PLAN

white bread
pies and cakes
ice cream
candy
doughnuts
honey (except for flavoring, and limit to one spoonful)
avocado
gravy
jelly and jam
marmalade
nuts
oil
peanut butter
potatoes
puddings
salad dressings (except as given later)
alcohol of any kind, including wine and beer

■ ■ ■

## HIGH-POWER REDUCING VEGETABLES TO ADD VARIETY TO YOUR MEALS WHILE DIETING

The following vegetables may be eaten during this 7-day reducing diet, for they are all in the category of the reducing-type of vegetables that take more calories to digest than they give to the body. You may continue to eat two or three bowls of the reducing soup whenever you feel hungry between meals, and then add variety to your lunches and dinners by using the following vegetables.

| | |
|---|---|
| string beans | asparagus |
| broccoli | brussels sprouts |
| cabbage | lettuce |
| celery | garlic |
| lettuce | kohlrabi |
| cucumbers | leeks |
| okra | mushrooms |
| green peppers | dill pickles |
| radishes | spinach |
| watercress | turnips |
| tomatoes | sauerkraut |

While on your reducing food plan you can eat any of the vegetables that grow above ground except peas, corn, and white beans. The only reason these are restricted while on the reducing food plan is that they are heavy in starches and carbohydrates. Later, when on the sustaining diet, these may be added to the regular diet in small quantities.

■ ■ ■

## ONE WOMAN LOST TEN POUNDS THE FIRST WEEK ON THIS DIET

Arline T. used this basic reducing plan. She did the two-day fasting diet first and immediately lost four pounds. Of course this was mostly water, but water adds up to pounds on your bathroom scales and also shows as puffiness on the body. Then Arline went on the actual Oriental diet of rice and vegetables, with a small piece of lean meat daily for only one week. At the end of that time she had lost the full ten pounds she desired! She did not want to lose more than the ten pounds, but when she saw with what ease she could, at will, remove the unwanted pounds, Arline lost her fear of dieting and the psychological shock that comes from the belief that we can do nothing to get rid of excessive weight.

From that time on Arline went on her sustaining diet, and she was able to keep her weight constantly at the level she desired. She felt so good on the rice, vegetables, fruits, grains, and a little meat, that she persisted in eating the rice long after she had lost her excess weight. She said the rice, eaten at least once daily, seemed to cushion her desire to eat big meals, and it also gave her a feeling of being full constantly. Arline also found that the rice satisfied her hunger urge to such an extent that it seemed to substitute for the candies, cakes, ice cream, and other carbohydrates that had wrecked her diet before. Rice satisfied the carbohydrate craving without adding the dangerous pounds of the other forms of starches, sugars, and carbohydrates.

Arline learned how to prepare rice in various ways, which I shall give later, and she even used rice for some delicious desserts.

■ ■ ■

## RESULTS YOU CAN EXPECT

At the end of the seven-day reducing period, you should actually have lost anywhere from ten to fifteen pounds. The amount varies with different people, for much depends on whether you are extremely active or whether you sit and rest a good deal. If you combine exercise with this Oriental diet, you can easily shed as much as fourteen pounds in that seven-day period. This is actually all that most people need to lose to get down to their ideal weight, but there are cases where one needs to lose from twenty to fifty pounds. What then?

If you find that you need to lose more weight after the seven-day period, you can extend this diet to another seven days, always limiting it to one week. This avoids the psychological block that most people face when they must diet over a prolonged period of time. It is like the alcoholic's pledge to stop drinking for only one day at a time.

A case from my files shows how a person can shed more than 50 pounds very easily on this Oriental reducing diet. Mrs. B. had continued to gain weight over the years until she tipped the scales at 185 pounds. Her normal weight for years had been 130 pounds.

She was now 45 years of age, and she was feeling fatigue and had symptoms of high blood pressure and other ailments that caused her doctor to tell her she should go on a stringent reducing diet. However, he did not recommend a particular diet.

As Mrs. B. was one of my lecture members, she asked my advice, and I gave her the complete Oriental diet system. The first two days, after fasting, she found she had lost 4 pounds. This, of course, was mostly water. But it encouraged her. When she began the actual reducing diet she suffered no hardships, for she found she did not miss the cakes, starches, sugars and carbohydrates she had taken daily for some years. The rice gave her a comfortably full feeling. The dieting soup satisfied her hunger pangs between meals, and in the first week of her diet she shed 14 pounds. This was so encouraging that she was able to easily extend her diet to another seven-day period. In this week she got rid of 20 more pounds. She kept the diet up for two more weeks, and easily lost the other 14 pounds and was down to her normal weight of 130 pounds. She was able to wear some of her former dresses, and the doctor told her when he examined her that her blood pressure was now normal and her heart action was improved over the time when she weighed 185 pounds. But the greatest benefits came in her relationships with her family and her husband. She now had the vitality and energy to enjoy her life and do her normal work without fatigue and boredom.

You can actually follow this Oriental reducing plan for several weeks and not be undernourished or suffer from hunger pangs, until you have lost your desired weight. Then if you should start to overeat again, and get back five or ten pounds, you can go back immediately on the 7-day diet until you are back to a normal weight once more.

Later in this book, you will be given many delicious recipes for preparing vegetables Oriental style, which will give you a wide variety of different dishes to serve with your meals, not only while you are losing weight pleasantly but when you go on the sustaining diet and wish to keep your weight at a fixed level.

You will also not be denied desserts, for I shall give you many fascinating Oriental desserts, utilizing the natural fruits that can give your sweet tooth a chance to be satisfied without taking into your body dangerous white sugars, white denatured flour, and the starches that we find in most American desserts and that are quickly turned into stored fat by the body!

# CHAPTER 3

# EAT FOR ENJOYMENT AS WELL AS FOR HEALTH

■ ■ ■

Eating should be enjoyable, not just for purposes of maintaining the body in good health. In any form of dieting many people lose sight of this fact. They go into various diets with a do-or-die determination that often robs them of one of life's greatest joys.

When you have attained the desired weight through my Oriental miracle diet, you face the problem of maintaining that weight and yet, at the same time, enjoying your food and not feeling that you are a slave to the system that keeps you slender but deprives you of one of life's greatest pleasures—eating.

There are many variations to this diet and many foods that you can continue to eat while on your sustaining diet, which will not only keep the pounds from ever coming back but will give you adequate nourishment and at the same time supply your taste buds with a pleasurable sensation that makes you feel you are really enjoying your food.

In this chapter we shall investigate some of these foods that may be eaten to vary the Oriental diet and that you will also require to keep the pounds off on your sustaining diet.

■ ■ ■

## THE DIFFERENCE BETWEEN CARBOHYDRATE FOODS AND PROTEIN FOODS

There is one important difference between carbohydrate foods and protein foods—it is chiefly one of taste. Carbohydrates are enjoyable to your taste buds because they are sweet. But the carbohydrates are dangerous if overused, because they are quickly converted into fat. The trick in any sustaining diet, after you have lost the desired number of pounds, is to substitute high-protein foods for the carbohydrates that you formerly ate and that brought back your weight quickly after dieting.

High-protein foods not only give you better nutrition than carbohydrate foods but they also give pleasure to your taste buds. They also tend to give you a feeling of being well fed, controlling your hunger thermostat, which makes you constantly crave sugars, starches, and carbohydrates. On these high-protein sustaining foods your body will actually be better nourished, and the extra pounds you worked hard to get rid of will not come back quickly.

You may still maintain a brown rice diet, but now, after losing the desired pounds, if you wish to retain your present desirable weight, eat the following foods, with the addition of the reducing vegetables given elsewhere.

A normal portion of these meats may be eaten, always broiled, boiled, or fried without fat in a Teflon pan:

Ground beef with all fat removed
Steaks, with fat trimmed off
Chicken, broiled or baked, with skin removed
Turkey, also with skin removed

Leg of lamb, baked
Veal

In addition to the above meats, which furnish the body with adequate protein, you should also vary the diet by including in your sustaining diet some of the following organ meats. Not only are these economical, but they contain valuable nutrients often not found in more popular cuts of meat.

Beef or calf's liver (calf's liver is more expensive and yet no more
    nutritional than the cheaper beef liver)
Kidneys
Hearts
Brains (these may be added to scrambled eggs and make an excel-
    lent breakfast or luncheon dish. A little butter may be used
    to cook them.)
Sweetbreads

During your actual seven-day reducing period avoid all pork products, but these may be added in small quantities after the desired weight has been lost. You can then eat bacon, which has been thoroughly cooked, thus removing most of the fat. It must be remembered any form of pork that is higher in caloric content than other meats are. For instance, there are three times more calories in one-half pound of pork sausage than in one-half pound of round steak. If you eat pork products, even on your sustaining diet, you face a risk of increasing your calories to a level that may bring back the pounds you have lost in dieting.

Also on the prohibited list while you are on your seven-day reducing diet are such foods as frankfurters, knockwurst, liverwurst, and other processed meats. After you have lost the desired weight, however, you may eat small portions of these products without fear.

You may eat fish during the diet period and after. Fish is one of the finest forms of protein and has an advantage over meat in that it has less fat. Shrimp, lobster, crab, canned tuna, and canned salmon may be added to your diet for variety while you are on the 7-day Oriental diet. Then when you are on your sustaining diet you may increase the portions. The fish can be eaten with vegetables or brown rice, or by itself.

Shrimp, crab, and lobster may be added to tasty cold salads, with a nonfattening dressing (to be given later). Or you may bake or broil other forms of fish. You should avoid fried fish, even on the sustaining diet, for it becomes saturated with fat, which adds to the calories. After all a total, daily caloric intake of 2,500 for women and about 3,200 for men is required to keep the body at its normal weight; any intake beyond these limits is bound to bring the fat back quickly. However we do not worry about calories while on the reducing 7-day Oriental diet because you can hardly eat more than 1,000 calories a day no matter how much you eat of the reducing soup, the vegetables, and the proteins given in this diet. We shall later have something to say about when calories do count in maintaining normal weight and when it becomes vitally important to know about the effects of exercise and the caloric requirements for various types of workers and those who lead sedentary lives.

You may also eat every type of cheese in small portions during dieting and afterward on your sustaining diet to maintain your normal weight. Dairy products are helpful in obtaining your required daily amounts of protein. Include cottage cheese, pot cheese, processed cheeses, and yogurt. You may drink skim milk, two glasses a day, and also use it in cooking various desserts, including rice pudding and custard. Eggs also make a good variation to meat protein intake. Later I shall give you some delicious recipes that can make eggs more tasty and nourishing than the usual frying, poaching, or boiling.

The above-mentioned protein foods are valuable in any diet plan, for they give you that variety that makes you feel you are eating all you wish, yet with the sure knowledge that these foods will give you a balanced diet and will keep the unwanted pounds off in the future.

After you have lost your undesired pounds you have to be eternally vigilant that you do not allow yourself to become careless in your sustaining diet and eat an excess of fat-producing carbohydrate foods, as the following case from my files illustrates.

Louise L. was a young schoolteacher whose weight was 155 pounds when she started the 7-day Oriental diet. She wanted to lose 25 pounds to be back to her normal 130 pounds. She began the diet, and it took her three weeks to lose the excess poundage, for she did not follow the diet too rigidly. But after the three weeks she was delighted that she no longer had to watch her weight so carefully, so she began to go back to her former diet. Soon the scales were tipping dangerously in the vicinity of 140 pounds. Louise then realized it was time to do something drastic. It was at this time that she consulted me.

I found out that Louise was making the old mistakes that had kept the fat on her body before. She was eating about 2,700 calories a day, mostly fat-producing foods, high in carbohydrates.

For breakfast she ate a dish of popular-brand cereal with milk and sugar. She had two cups of coffee, with cream and sugar. She also had a glass of orange juice and two slices of white toast with butter.

Louise's lunch usually consisted of a piece of fried or broiled meat; sometimes a hamburger, with cheese and on a white bun. She varied this luncheon at times with macaroni, and occasionally with her hamburger she had French-fried potatoes and topped it off with a malt, or a piece of pie or cake, and another cup of coffee with cream and sugar!

You can well understand why Louise was soon right back where she started on this vicious cycle of overindulgence of fattening foods. To make matters worse, at dinner she ate another meat dish, with vegetables flavored with butter, and again a carbohydrate dessert of ice cream, Jello, cake, or something equally fattening, and with another cup of coffee and cream.

On this diet Louise was eating more than 3,000 calories a day, and these were fat calories—that is, fat-producing foods. She actually needed only about 2,000 calories a day for her work schedule, for she did little physical work. During the reducing diet with the Oriental system, she actually consumed about 1,200 calories a day, which was one of the reasons why her weight loss was gradual.

The moment Louise discovered that her weight was coming back rapidly she became most discouraged. When she consulted me I told her that even on her sustaining diet she must eat fewer carbohydrates and proteins than she was. In fact, she had to keep her daily caloric intake to about 2,000 calories a day or the weight would come back rapidly.

Louise began a sustaining diet that included the following foods. For breakfast:

2 boiled eggs
A small glass orange juice or one-half of a grapefruit
1 slice of dry, slightly hard, whole-wheat toast
Ovaltine with soymilk and $1/4$ tsp. pure maple syrup

For lunch Louise could still have a portion of lean meat which could be veal, beef, or chicken, broiled or cooked without fat. She could eat no more than two of the vegetables that grow above the ground, such as corn or peas, that are not listed on the 7-day-diet group of vegetables. She could vary this with any other vegetables she wished on other days. No bread or butter was permitted at lunch, but she could eat a bowlfull of brown rice flavored with butter, and have a glass of skim milk, with her sugarless Jello or fruit for dessert.

Now you can well see this was no starvation diet for Louise. Yet it was a sustaining diet that could keep her slender and at the same time furnish her with a balanced, nutrititious diet. For dinner I told Louise to eat a small bowl of the diet soup, to kill her appetite. This gave her bulk. Then she could eat a regular portion of ground beef, with fat removed and broiled, or fried without fat. Or she could vary this on some nights with a small salad, with lemon-and-oil dressing; and if she was still hungry (which was unlikely if she ate the vegetable soup), she could add one or two vegetables such as broccoli or asparagus tips, with a little melted butter. For dessert she could have a portion of fresh or canned fruit if the syrup was washed off.

The upshot of this new sustaining diet was that Louise was back to her normal 130 pounds within two weeks. From that time she simply maintained her regular sustaining diet, adding proteins instead of carbohydrates to her daily food intake, until she found the perfect diet to keep her at her desired weight.

■ ■ ■

## THE IMPORTANCE OF A GOOD BREAKFAST IN WEIGHT REDUCTION

Wake up, sleepyhead—it's time for breakfast! Common sense says so, medical research proves it, and your own body tells you that breakfast is the most important meal of the day. But many of us imagine ourselves as simply being too busy weekday mornings to pay much mind to something this necessary for good health.

Typical of most single- or two-parent households with kids is something like this: got to get the children up, the dog walked, the cat fed, the coffee made, the paper read, the lunches packed, myself washed and dressed and out the door on the way to work. Who has time anyway to eat breakfast, let alone cook it, you reason. Does any of this sound uncomfortably familiar, by chance?

A small, independent telephone survey of the country's breakfast habits sponsored by the Kellogg Co. did show that about 93 percent of American adults do eat at least one item in the morning. The telephone poll, surveying five hundred adults at random across the country, found the following to be the most common breakfast foods, ranked according to their popularity:

| | |
|---|---|
| Cold cereal with milk | 49% |
| Plain or buttered toast | 30% |
| Eggs/omelets with toast | 28% |
| Coffee or tea | 28% |
| A glass of juice | 23% |

While this may be less than the ideal of a nutritionally balanced breakfast, it is certainly better than going without eating anything.

But there are certain inherent dangers in allowing yourself either a skimpy breakfast too often or else ignoring it all together and going without *any* nourishment. Excessive caffeine on an empty stomach can increase the heart rate, overstimulate the nerves, and elevate blood pressure. According to work done by cardiologist Renata Cifkova, people who shun breakfast and opt for coffee or tea instead may spend their mornings at higher risk of heart problems, including heart attacks. This is according to information that appeared in *Science News* (130:246) for April 20, 1991.

Another potentially serious health problem that results from skipping breakfast is a sudden drop in blood sugar level. Such diet-imposed hypoglycemia can lead to a sudden loss of energy, immediate fatigue, incoherent behavior, and faulty thinking. Caffeine is known to reduce body blood sugar, and the addition of fruit juices early in the morning on an empty stomach only makes matters worse. Athletes are especially guilty of this, noted the July 1992 issue of *The Physician and Sportsmedicine* (20[7]:29).

But the best news yet in favor of eating a well-balanced breakfast is that it will help to control your weight. By eating something every morning before you start your day's activities, you will reduce impulsive snacking habits that usually lead to unwanted weight gain. According to the March 1992 issue of *The American Journal of Clinical Nutrition* (55[3]:645), eating breakfast can help you to lose a "significant" amount of weight.

Researchers studied fifty-two overweight women aged eighteen to fifty-five and assigned them to a weight-loss program for twelve weeks. They were divided into two groups. One was the no-breakfast group, whose members ate only two meals a day, and the other was the breakfast group, whose members ate three meals a day.

The results of the study indicated that those who ate breakfast had a lower fat intake and a much higher carbohydrate intake than those who did not eat breakfast. Another advantage was that breakfast eaters ate fewer impulsive snacks and reduced the fats and calories that are associated with them.

Apparently, eating breakfast helps reduce impulsive snacking throughout the day and, therefore, could play a major role in weight loss overall. Nutrition experts think that breakfast is a vital part of a healthy diet. But in spite of this sound advice, nearly 40 percent of women aged twenty-five to thirty-four routinely miss eating something in the morning.

Others follow the mistaken logic that forgoing breakfast will help them lose weight because their calorie intake will be less. Nothing could be further from the truth. To the contrary, scientists state that eating breakfast foods helps to keep a person from overeating the rest of the day.

Skipping breakfast appears to be associated with overeating at other meals or with increased between-meal snacking. This in turn always leads to a higher overall intake of calories, and thus a gradual gain in weight.

The bottom line here seems to be that if you're desperately trying to lose weight but not experiencing much success, then breakfast just might be your best friend. Researchers recommend that you include a low-fat, high-carbohydrate breakfast as part of your weight-loss program. For instance, this might include whole-grain cereals with skim milk, bagels, or English muffins. But more about what it takes to build a good breakfast a bit later.

New research underscored the importance not only of breakfast itself, but also of the *type* of food consumed in relationship to hunger later in the day. In a short-term study at the Minneapolis Veterans Administration Medical Center, thirty-three healthy adults, twenty-four to fifty-nine years of age, were randomly assigned various meals for breakfast. None had eaten since 10 P.M. the previous night. The results were briefly highlighted in an edition of the *New York Times* for Wednesday, May 23, 1990 (p. B6).

At 7:30 A.M. some participants ate cereal with no fiber; others ate cereal with 11 grams of fiber per serving. At 11 A.M. all the participants were offered an unlimited buffet. Then the researchers measured the food intake and surveyed the participants regarding the amount of food they ate at breakfast and lunch as well as how hungry they felt before the buffet.

What they learned was that eating a high-fiber cereal helped the participants slash 150 calories or more from their breakfast and lunch intakes. This was in part because high-fiber cereals contain fewer calories per serving, and in part because fiber can decrease the appetite.

There are several theories about the relationship between fiber and appetite. First, fiber may slow the rate at which the stomach empties. Second, when fiber reaches the colon it ferments and produces a feeling of fullness. The products of fermentation, like fatty acids, can decrease the appetite. Finally, the fiber in whole-grain cereals produces more gas, which may also diminish appetite.

The late Robert Rodale (whose father founded Rodale Press and *Prevention* health magazine many years ago) understood the value of a good breakfast. Not only did it give him boundless energy for a hectic day, but it also *kept him slender* throughout all of his adult life! The following information has been compiled from his book *Sane Living in a Mad World* (Emmaus, PA: Rodale Press, 1972, pp. 149–155).

He called breakfast "my number-one health secret!" He gave a couple of very logical reasons why eating something in the morning is so vital for good health. He believed that the body should be fresh and rested by then, thus, the work of digestion wouldn't tire the body as much then as it would later in the day.

He then let readers in on his little health secret. "My habit is to eat a breakfast so big that I sometimes feel slightly stuffed for a few minutes afterward. But I can digest all that food easily in the morning, and the rest of the day I have *less* desire to eat. I coast along all day on that big breakfast, satisfied and with plenty of energy."

Rodale offered some good tips for *wanting* to eat a good breakfast—not something everyone is willing to get into the habit of doing. "You have to look at the day as a twenty-four-hour entity," he wrote. "Think of *when* you are going to want to be the most active, *when* you need the fuel and energy of a good meal, *when* your body is going to be in the best condition to do the work of digestion." By looking at breakfast in those terms, he advised, "you'll probably see what is obvious to me—daylight is the time you need the energy." So, he continued this train of thought by reiterating his point, that eating a good meal *before* starting the day is the most logical thing to do.

But looking at the entire day is valuable for still another reason, he argued. "You can't isolate breakfast. If you're going to eat a larger meal in the morning, you'll have to cut down elsewhere to finish the day with the same or fewer calories." He then summed up what he meant. "When I say, 'Eat a big breakfast,' I am really saying, 'Eat a big breakfast, and eat a little less for lunch and supper.'" But more important to him was what is consumed *after* dinner. "Eating in the evening is fatal to the desire for a good meal in the morning. If you go to bed with a snack-filled stomach, you won't feel much like eating in the morning."

Robert Rodale made as the cornerstones of his breakfast menu the following items:

Cooked cornmeal mush
Whole-grain toast with old-fashioned peanut butter
Buckwheat pancakes with pure maple syrup
Cooked oatmeal

His own "cereal" creation: equal parts of cracked sunflower and pumpkin seeds, wheat germ, apple or banana flakes, raisins and dried skim milk powder

Fruit (such as an apple, banana, some berries, a melon, and even dried fruit)

He had some final words to say about eggs. He mentioned that the media have routinely presented information to the effect that eggs are bad to eat, simply because they're high in cholesterol. While this may be the case, it certainly doesn't justify omitting them altogether from your breakfast, he argued. "Eggs are most pleasant eating, and they are an excellent source of the protein we need in the morning," he wrote. "The content of cholesterol is largely counteracted by the lecithin they contain. The whole cholesterol question is one of common sense. If we eat foods that are natural, wholesome and unprocessed, we are almost bound to have a good diet."

He bragged about eating two eggs almost every day of his life. And that the last time he had a blood workup done for a check on his cholesterol level, it was a healthy 176 milligrams per deciliter of blood. But he also was quick to point out that he didn't eat other things with his eggs that might have sent his serum cholesterol soaring, items such as ham, bacon, butter, cream, or sugar.

A final observation he made in relation to eating a good-sized breakfast every morning: He stated that he ate a much lighter lunch than most people would (somewhere around 2 p.m.) and that his evening meals were often "quite small." Most of his health philosophy correlates nicely with the eating patterns of most people throughout the Orient. Over the past quarter-century I've traveled to most of the countries lining the Pacific Rim and have discovered just how true this is with the common working classes. The only exception to this are the high-powered lunches and dinners of some Korean or Japanese businessmen. Otherwise, the majority of people make breakfast one of their most important meals, to start their days off right.

■ ■ ■

## BUILDING GREAT BREAKFASTS THAT FILL YOU UP BUT *NOT* OUT

The previous chapter provided extensive information about the value of rice in a weight-loss diet. One of the main reasons that rice works so well at breakfast time is that it can fill you up but not out. Put another way, hunger is satisfied, energy reserves are increased, but no extra weight is put on.

One half of this planet's entire population subsists on rice. In Asia alone, an estimated six hundred pounds of rice is consumed per person every year. This is an astonishing figure when you realize that is reduced to a daily consumption of about one and a half pounds per individual per day.

No one seems to eat more rice per meal than the people of the Orient. Now wonder that the vast majority of them are so slender. Yet at the same time they're also very energetic. To understand what rice has accomplished in terms of human strength and endurance, just look at the Great Wall of northern China. It is the only man-made object on earth that the astronauts can clearly see from outer space without the aid of a telescope! It is a long, winding affair of some fifteen hundred miles, running mostly along the southern edge of the Mongolian plain, from the Kansu Province to the Hopeh Province on the Yellow Sea. The wall was erected to protect China from northern nomads. Millions of laborers were conscripted from all over China to help build it. Their principal food was lots and lots of steamed rice, morning, noon, and night! Now if that isn't a testimony to the marvelous nutritive powers of rice, then I'd like to know just what is.

Here are some suggestions for assembling good breakfasts that will give you loads of energy without pounds of fat. Since the theme of this book is geared toward Oriental health secrets for quick and efficient weight loss, it is only fitting to start out with some rice breakfast dishes. I am indebted to Marie Simmons, a food writer and recipe developer from Brooklyn, New York, for the first several recipes, which have been somewhat revised to fit the theme of this chapter, namely, to eat well for fun and well-being.

## BREAKFAST RICE PUDDING

$1/2$ cup uncooked long-grain white rice

$1/4$ cup pure maple syrup

$1/4$ tsp. salt

$1/4$ tsp. ground cinnamon

2 qts. goat milk (canned or packaged, if necessary)

$1/4$ cup raisins

$1/2$ cup lichee nuts, drained and chopped

Preheat the oven to 325°F. Combine the rice, syrup, salt, and cinnamon in a large shallow $2^1/2$ qt. baking dish. Stir in 1 quart of goat's milk until thoroughly blended. (*Note:* Soymilk may be substituted, if desired.)

Place the baking dish on the center rack of the oven. Gradually stir in the remaining quart of milk and bake for $2^1/2$ hours, stirring once after the first half hour. After 1 hour of baking stir the brown edges into the pudding several times. Stir the raisins and lichee nuts in after 2 hours, then bake undisturbed for the final $1/2$ hour until a top crust forms.

Set on a wire rack and cool. Makes an excellent breakfast dish. If you desire a pudding with a little crunch to it, then stir in a little granola, some broken pieces of rice cake, or slivers of crushed nuts with the raisins and lichee nuts. Yields about 9 servings.

## BANANA RICE PUDDING

4 extra-large, farm-fresh egg yolks

$1/2$ cup honey

2 cups soymilk (mixed according to directions on package label)

2 cups cooked long-grain white rice

$^1/_4$ cup plain yogurt

1 tsp. pure vanilla extract

$^1/_2$ cup mashed medium-ripe banana

1 cup sliced medium-ripe banana

Ground cinnamon

In a large bowl whisk the egg yolks and honey thoroughly. Meanwhile, heat the soymilk in a medium-sized saucepan until nearly boiling. Gradually whisk the hot milk into the egg yolks until completely blended.

Pour this mixture back into the saucepan. Cook over low heat, stirring often, until the mixture starts to thicken and eventually coats a metal spoon (about 12 minutes). Stir in the rice and cook over low heat, stirring, until very thick, about 6 minutes. Stir in the yogurt. Let stand off the heat, stirring frequently, for 5 minutes, then add the vanilla as you continue to stir.

Pour everything into a bowl and refrigerate until well chilled. Just before eating prepare the bananas. First stir in the mashed banana until well blended; then fold in the sliced banana. Spoon some of this into a small bowl and sprinkle with ground cinnamon before enjoying. Yields 6 servings.

### CHINESE HOT RICE WITH FRUIT AND HONEY

1 cup uncooked long-grain white rice

$2^1/_4$ cups water

$^1/_4$ cup dried apricot or apple, or the equivalent in cut-up fruit leather

1 Tbsp. unsalted butter

$^1/_4$ tsp. salt

$1^1/_2$ cups plain yogurt

honey to taste

ground nutmeg

fresh, sliced lichee nuts

Combine the rice, water, dried fruit, butter, and salt in a medium-sized saucepan. Heat over low heat until boiling, stirring until the rice is tender and the water is absorbed (this should take about 17 minutes).

Next add the yogurt and cook over low heat, stirring, until the rice is thick and creamy, about 5 minutes. Then spoon some into a bowl and drizzle with honey in a spiraling motion. Sprinkle with a pinch of powdered nutmeg and top with sliced lichee nuts. Yields 4 servings.

## Brown Rice with Nuts and Raisins

2 cups cooked short- or long-grain brown rice

2 cups goat milk or soymilk

$1/4$ cup raisins

1 Tbsp. broken almonds

1 Tbsp. broken cashews

1 tsp. unsalted butter (optional)

1 Tbsp. honey

Combine the rice and milk in a medium-sized saucepan and heat to boiling. Cook over medium heat, stirring, until the mixture thickens, about 12 minutes. Stir in the raisins and cook for an additional 3 minutes.

Then spoon some of this into a bowl and sprinkle it with the broken pieces of both nutmeats. Add a little pat of butter, if desired, and then stir in the honey. Yields 4 servings.

Stephanie Simmons came up with this nifty breakfast dish that is fast and easy to fix.

## Hot Oatmeal and Rice Cereal

1 cup water

$1/2$ cup regular-cut oatmeal

$1/2$ cup leftover cooked white or brown rice

1 Tbsp. raisins

Pure maple syrup

In a small saucepan heat the water to boiling. Then stir in the oatmeal and cook, stirring, for about 4 minutes. Add the rice and cook, stirring, until the mixture thickens. Stir in the raisins next. Spoon into a bowl and stir in some maple syrup from Vermont or eastern Canada. Yields 1 serving.

### Wellness Flapjacks

If you want a low-fat, high-fiber breakfast that's also tasty and festive, pancakes may be just be the ticket. Pancakes made from mixes usually derive 20 percent to 35 percent of their calories from fat—or even less if you use 2 percent milk and only a small amount of oil. But complete mixes, to which you add only water, usually contain partially hydrogenated oils as well as whole milk. Most mixes contain little cholesterol, but if eggs are called for, you may use them without feeling guilty (remember Robert Rodale's comments).

The real problem, though, with most pancake mixes in not so much high fat and cholesterol but a great deal of sodium—almost 900 milligrams per serving in some instances—from added salt and leavening agents such as sodium aluminum phosphate and baking soda. Another potential problem is the hefty amount of butter and syrup most folks like to put on top of their hotcakes.

If you think your pancakes need more fiber, you may add any of the following to the batter: wheat bran or germ, oat bran, rice bran, instant oatmeal, diced apples, blueberries, or even grated carrots.

Pancakes are strictly an American thing, of course, and really have nothing to do with the Orient. But they fit in with this diet for a couple of reasons. First and most importantly, they fill you up so you won't be so tempted to snack in between meals. Second, flapjacks are a very popular American food—people of all ages everywhere seem to enjoy them. And third, they are very easy to make. For ten pancakes combine $1^1/_2$ cups of white or whole wheat flour, 1 tsp. of baking powder, $^1/_2$ tsp. baking soda, 2 egg whites, $^1/_2$ cup plain nonfat yogurt, $^1/_2$ cup 2 percent milk, and 1 Tbsp. of vegetable oil. Thin the batter with more milk, if necessary. You can also substitute 2 percent milk or buttermilk for the yogurt if you wish. (But the acidity of soured dairy products adds a nice flavor and makes the hotcakes rise better.) Use a nonstick pan or griddle, coated or sprayed with a little bit of oil. Use about two heaping tablespoons of batter for each pancake.

### *Healthful Pancake Toppings*

Most pancakes syrups have somewhere between 100 and 135 calories per two-tablespoon serving. Honey has 130 calories per two tablespoons, and so does maple syrup. So-called "lite" syrups are diluted with water, and thus have about 50 calories per serving. Some syrups contain 100 milligrams of sodium per serving. For a syrup that is virtually sodium-free, always be sure to use pure maple syrup.

For a deliciously sweet syrup with half the calories of honey, thaw $1/2$ a cup of frozen apple juice concentrate and mix it with 2 Tbsp. of apple cider or water.

Consider other toppings, too, alone or combined with a little syrup: cooked or fresh fruit and berries, or fruit conserves. Chunky apples stewed in apple juice and flavored with cinnamon are very good also.

A tablespoon of butter adds 100 calories and 12 grams of artery-clogging fat. People who skip it say the pancakes taste just as good. You should never use margarine, as it is very unhealthful for you.

### *Rise and Shine: Flavorful Breakfast Treats on the Lean Side*

The French toast recipe that follows was contributed by Elaine Michura of Chicago, Illinois and the muffin recipe by Constance O'Toole of Barrington, Rhode Island, and Sue Covelle of Malden, Massachusetts. The recipes have been revised in a test kitchen to remove almost 20 grams of fat per serving. While slimmed down, there has nonetheless been no loss of flavor.

#### DIETER'S FRENCH TOAST

1 large egg

2 large egg whites

$3/4$ cup skim milk

2 Tbsp. brown sugar

1 tsp. pure vanilla extract

$1/4$ tsp. ground cinnamon

$^1/_8$ tsp. baking powder

8 $^1/_2$-inch-thick slices Italian bread

2 tsp. sunflower or sesame seed oil

1 tsp. butter

### THE SYRUP

$^1/_2$ cup sugar

$^1/_4$ cup dark corn syrup

$^1/_2$ tsp. ground cinnamon

$^1/_4$ cup water

$^1/_4$ cup evaporated skim milk

*French toast preparation:* In a medium-sized bowl, whisk together egg, egg whites, milk, sugar, vanilla, cinnamon, and baking powder until well blended. Place the bread slices in a large, shallow baking dish and pour egg mixture over the top; turn to coat evenly. Press a piece of wax paper directly on the bread to cover it, then cover the dish with plastic wrap. Refrigerate overnight.

Next morning, heat 1 tsp. of the oil and $^1/_2$ tsp. of the butter in a 12-inch nonstick skillet over medium-high heat. Add four of the soaked bread slices to the pan and cook until golden on both sides, 2 to 3 minutes per side. Transfer the toast to a platter and keep warm in a warm oven. Cook the remaining slices in the same manner, using the remaining 1 tsp. oil and $^1/_2$ tsp. butter. Yields 4 servings.

*Syrup preparation:* In a small saucepan, stir together the sugar, corn syrup, cinnamon, and water. Bring the mixture to a boil over medium-high heat, stirring constantly. Boil for 2 minutes. Remove from heat and stir in evaporated skim milk. Let cool; transfer to a small pitcher. (*Note:* This syrup can be stored, covered in the refrigerator, for up to 7 days. If desired, warm before serving.)

## HALLELUJAH MUFFINS

$1^1/_2$ cups all-purpose white flour

$^1/_2$ cup whole-wheat flour

$1^1/_4$ cups sugar

1 Tbsp. ground cardamom

1 tsp. baking powder

1 tsp. baking soda

$^1/_2$ tsp. salt

2 cups grated carrots (4 medium)

1 apple, peeled, cored, and chopped (1 cup)

1 cup raisins

1 large egg, lightly beaten

2 large egg whites, lightly beaten

$^1/_2$ cup apple butter

$^1/_4$ sunflower or sesame seed oil

1 Tbsp. pure vanilla extract

2 Tbsp. finely chopped walnuts

2 Tbsp. toasted wheat germ

Preheat the oven to 375°F. Lightly oil 18 muffin cups. In a large bowl, stir together flours, sugar, cardamom, baking powder, baking soda, and salt. Stir in carrots, apple, and raisins. In a medium-sized bowl, whisk together the eggs, egg whites, apple butter, oil, and vanilla. Add to the dry ingredients and stir just until moistened.

Then spoon the batter into the prepared muffin cups, filling them about three quarters full. In a small bowl, combine the walnuts and wheat germ; sprinkle these over the muffin tops. Bake for 17 minutes or until tops are golden and spring back when lightly pressed. Yields 18 muffins.

### "Awful" Waffles a "Neat" Treat

This recipe with the clever name and great taste came from Pam Sturges of Cincinnati, Ohio.

1 cup whole-wheat flour

1 cup all-purpose white flour

$1^1/_4$ tsp. baking powder

$^1/_2$ tsp. baking soda

Pinch of salt

2 cups buttermilk

1 large egg

1 Tbsp. rum extract

1 Tbsp. sesame seed oil, plus extra for preparing the waffle iron

2 egg whites

2 Tbsp. brown sugar

In a large bowl, stir together both kinds of flour, the baking powder, and baking soda. In a separate bowl, whisk together the buttermilk, egg, rum extract, and oil. Add to the dry ingredients and stir with a wooden spoon until moistened.

In a mixing bowl, beat the 2 egg whites with an electric mixer until soft peaks form. Add the brown sugar and continue beating until stiff and glossy. Whisk one quarter of the beaten egg whites into the batter. With a rubber spatula, fold in the remaining beaten egg whites.

Preheat the waffle iron. Brush the surface lightly with oil. Fill the iron two thirds full. Cook for 5–6 minutes, or until the waffles are crisp and golden. Repeat with the remaining batter, brushing the surface with oil before cooking each batch. Yields about 6 waffles.

■ ■ ■

## THE "POWER" LUNCH FOR STAYING SLIM

The next most important meal in our daily diets is lunch. Harvey A. Levenstein, a professor of history at McMaster University in Hamilton,

Ontario, gave a brief background regarding the evolution of lunch in the United States in his fascinating book *Revolution at the Table: The Transformation of the American Diet* (New York: Oxford University Press, 1988).

The first hot lunches that were served quickly over counters were set up in railway stations in the eastern United States in the beginning of the 1880s. A decade and a half later the first cafeteria opened in Chicago and offered an expanded variety of lunches. By the first decade of the twentieth century, swelling numbers of office workers had stimulated the establishment of many such restaurants for the noonday crowd. Before Prohibition, many cafeterias met stiff competition for the masculine trade from the saloon's "free lunch" (Rarely were these lunches free, but they cost only a nominal amount, usually a nickel or so). But following Prohibition the way was opened for a greater expansion in restaurants catering to the lunch-hour trade. About this time the four- or five-course "businessman's lunch" came into being and remained with slight changes for a number of decades thereafter.

With the advent of World War II and a dramatic increase in America's industrialization, several million factory workers found themselves packing lunches that were mostly made up of cheap meat or peanut-butter-and-jelly sandwiches and thermos jugs full of coffee. The twelve o'clock ritual for many blue-collar laborers had become a time for the consumption of inexpensive fare designed primarily with the intention of filling them up. Little thought was ever given to just how unhealthful such artery-clogging foods were. As a result the incidence of cancer, heart disease, obesity, and other diet-related illnesses started to climb in America.

With the dawn of the health food movement sometime in the early 1970s, some Americans began taking serious charge of their own health. As more information became available in the popular press, people started changing to healthier lifestyles. They exercised more, ate better, and learned new ways to relax. Evident among these gradual improvements were significant changes in the way they ate lunch. Red meat was out and chicken and fish were in. Real men (and women) began eating more quiche, and suddenly salads became the rage for maintaining normal weight. The next two decades saw a more diet-conscious America eating avocado sandwiches, slurping down lentil soup, and sipping herbal teas. At least, that is, the better-educated and economically advantaged were doing this. Vegetarianism was no longer a kooky way of eating; by now it had become a sensible alternative to the simultaneously burgeoning fast-food industry, with its greasy burgers, fries, and chicken, and colas, soft drinks, and milkshakes.

To stay healthy and keep your weight under control, it is imperative that you pay more attention to what you eat *at noontime*. The importance of breakfast and what constitutes a good one have already been discussed. Lunch is the next meal that requires close scrutiny. Those who've been successful losing weight and keeping it off with the Oriental 7-day diet know that giving careful thought to lunch is just as important as devoting attention to breakfast.

There is almost an endless variety of good things that can be easily prepared for a nourishing and tasty lunch. I've selected some of the best meal choices for your midday dining pleasure, meals that will keep your energy supply steadily flowing, but without packing your abdomen, hips, thighs, and buttocks with ugly and unwanted pounds. Some of these recipes have a definite Oriental flavor to them, while others could be described as being somewhat vegetarian. *Bon appetit!*

### BOILED WATERCRESS WITH CHINESE SAUCE

This is a popular dish with the noontime crowds in the capitol city of Taipei, Taiwan. The chef who furnished me the recipe (with the aid of an interpreter, of course) failed to include the exact proportions. But it is quite simple to make, and a little experimentation will get you the right ingredient amounts, depending on how much you wish to make.

Some water

Some watercress

A little soy sauce

Some sesame seed oil

Some Chinese rice vinegar

A little freshly ground black pepper

$1/_2$ of an onion, finely chopped

Cook the watercress in enough water to cover until tender. Strain and mix with soy sauce, sesame seed oil, vinegar, and a few grindings of black pepper to taste. Sprinkle raw onion on top and eat.

### LAMBS QUARTERS WITH MUSHROOMS

1 Tbsp. soy sauce

1 Tbsp. pale dry sherry

$1/2$ tsp. cornstarch

3 Tbsp. sesame seed oil

1 large clove garlic, finely chopped

1 scallion, including some green, finely chopped

$1/2$ tsp. fresh ginger root, peeled and finely chopped

$1/4$ cup fairy ring mushrooms (*Marasmius oreades*) wiped or washed and stems removed

2 cups (about 3 oz.) lambs quarters washed and coarsely chopped (tough stems should be removed)

$1/2$ cup water

In a small bowl combine the soy sauce, sherry, and cornstarch. Heat a 12-inch wok or iron skillet over a high burner for 30 seconds (if gas flame) or 5 minutes (if electric). Then add the oil and heat the cooking utensil another 30 seconds (for gas flame) or about 2 minutes (for electric). Add the garlic, scallion, ginger, and mushrooms, and stir-fry for 1 minute (3 minutes for electric). Add the lambs quarters and stir-fry for 3 minutes (6 minutes for electric). Next pour in the water and cook, covered, for 7 minutes, until the water is gone and the greens are tender.

Recombine the soy sauce, sherry, and cornstarch and pour over the greens. Mix well until the sauce thickens and serve. Yields 4 servings for a Chinese meal, but half that amount for Western-style lunch.

### AMARANTH WITH RICE STICK NOODLES

2 oz. rice stick noodles

$1^1/2$ Tbsp. soy sauce

1 tsp. sesame seed oil

2 Tbsp. pale dry sherry

$^1/_8$ tsp. hot sauce

3 Tbsp. water

3 Tbsp. sesame seed oil

1 large garlic clove, finely chopped

2 scallions, including some green, finely chopped

1 small zucchini, ends removed, scrubbed and sliced into
  julienne strips

1 cup (about $1^1/_2$ oz.) amaranth leaves and stems, washed and
  chopped medium fine

Soak the rice stick noodles in enough hot water to cover for 15
minutes. Cut them into 2-inch lengths. In a small bowl combine
the soy sauce, sesame seed oil, sherry, hot sauce, and water.
Then heat a 12-inch wok or iron skillet over a gas burner
(turned all the way up) for about 45 seconds. Add the rest of
the sesame oil and heat for another 25 seconds. Add the garlic
and scallions, mix, then add the zucchini and amaranth. Stir-fry
for about 4 minutes until the vegetables become tender. Mix in
the rice noodles and then add the bowl of seasoning mixture.
Bring to a boil and serve. This yields 4 servings for a Chinese
lunch, but only half this amount for a Western-style lunch.

I've made this myself sometimes when I've wanted a light lunch.
It is delicious, easily digestible, quite filling, and very healthful.

### PRESSED SALAD WITH PINE NUTS

1 head romaine lettuce

1 carrot

2 stalks celery

1 Tbsp. sea salt

$^1/_2$ cup pine nuts

Wash the lettuce, pat dry with paper towels, and shred the leaves
into a large wooden bowl. Wash the carrot but do not scrub it,
so that the minerals remain intact with the skin. Shred with a

hand grater and add to the lettuce; then chop the celery (leaves included) into small pieces and add to the mixture. Sprinkle the salad with salt and toss. Place a plate directly on top of the vegetables and put an 8- or 10-pound weight of some kind on top of the plate. Permit to stand like this for $1/2$ an hour.

Now pour off the water from the salad and lightly rinse away the salt if desired. Add the pine nuts and serve. (*Note:* If you suffer from hypertension, you may want to omit the salt.) Yields 4 servings.

## SQUASH AND ONIONS

1 butternut squash

3 medium yellow onions

1 Tbsp. sunflower seed oil

$1/2$ tsp. oregano

$1/2$ cup water

$1/4$ tsp. granulated kelp

Wash and scrub the squash; cut into 2-inch pieces. Peel the onions, cut in half lengthwise, then slice into $1/2$-inch-wide strips. Heat the oil in a 2-quart saucepan, add the onions, and sauté until transparent. Add the squash and oregano and sauté for another $2^1/2$ minutes. Then add the water and granulated kelp; reduce the heat, cover, and cook for almost $1/2$ hour. Yields 4 servings.

## STEAMED GARLIC BROCCOLI

1 bunch broccoli

1 clove garlic

$1/2$ cup water

Granulated kelp

Sunflower seeds, hulled

Wash and chop the broccoli, separating the stems and flowerettes; mince the garlic. Place the broccoli stems in a $1^1/2$-quart saucepan with the water and garlic; cover and steam for 4 minutes. Uncover and stir the stems; arrange the flowerettes on top, then cover and steam for another 4 minutes. Serve with granulated kelp and a light sprinkling of hulled sunflower seeds.

### SQUASH CREAM SOUP

3 cups leftover squash and onions

2 cups water

Pinch of sea salt

Chopped parsley

Puree vegetables and water in a Vita-Mix Total Nutrition Center (see Appendix II) until creamy. Then transfer to a soup pot and add the salt; heat thoroughly but don't allow to boil. Garnish with chopped parsley. Yields 4 servings.

### STRING BEANS TAHINI WITH KASHA

$1^1/_2$ lb. string beans

$^2/_3$ cup water

2 Tbsp. natural soy sauce (shoyu) to taste

4 Tbsp. tahini (nut butter made with white sesame seeds)

### KASHA

2 cups whole brown kasha (buckwheat groats)

$3^3/_4$ cups water

$^1/_2$ tsp. sea salt

Snap the ends off the beans, break them in half, and wash thoroughly. Place the beans in a 2- or 3-quart saucepan with water. Cover and simmer for 10 minutes. Add the soy sauce and cook for another 10 minutes. Then remove the beans from the heat and carefully blend in the tahini. (*Note:* Don't boil the tahini or it is apt to curdle.)

*Kasha:* Bring water to boil in a 2- or 3-quart pot. Add the kasha and salt, then reduce heat to a minimum. Cover and cook for 15 minutes or until fluffy. Spoon string bean mixture over individual servings of kasha and eat. Yields 4 servings.

## STEAMED COLLARD GREENS

1 bunch collard greens

Water

Sea salt to taste

1 bay leaf

Several drops of rice vinegar

Trim 2 to 3 inches from the collard stems and wash the leaves well. Slice twice lengthwise, then chop crosswise in thin pieces. Place the collard pieces, salt, and bay leaf in a 2- or 3-quart pot with $1/2$ inch water. Steam over low heat for 9 minutes. Add the rice vinegar during the last 2 minutes of cooking. Yields 4 servings.

## BOILED HONG KONG SALAD

$1/2$ cup onions, cut into thick half-moons

1 cup kale, sliced into $1^1/_2$-inch-wide pieces

$1/2$ cup carrots, cut into thin half-moons

1 cup cabbage, cut into 1-inch chunks

water

Place about an inch of water in a pot and bring to a boil. Boil the onions for about 1 minute. Use a slotted spoon or a pair of cooking chopsticks to remove onions, leaving cooking water in the pot. Drain onions in a colander before placing in a large serving bowl. Boil the kale in the same water for $1^1/_2$ minutes; remove and drain. Place in the bowl with the onions.

Then boil the carrots in the same water for $1^1/_2$ minutes. Remove the cooked carrots, drain, and mix in with the kale and onions. Finally, cook the cabbage in the boiling water for almost 2 minutes. Remove, drain, and mix in with the other vegetables. Serve plain or with equal parts of rice vinegar and olive oil (well shaken). Yields 2 servings.

### TOKYO LENTIL SOUP

$1/2$ cup lentils, washed

$1/4$ cup onions, diced

$1/4$ carrots, diced

$1/8$ cup celery, diced

1 strip kombu (a wide, dark-green, mineral-rich sea vegetable),
   $11/2$ inches long, soaked and diced

2–3 cups water

Pinch of sea salt

Place the lentils, onions, carrots, celery, kombu, and water in a pot and bring to a boil. Cover and reduce flame to low. Simmer about 45 minutes. Season with a very small amount of sea salt and simmer another 17 minutes until the lentils and vegetables are soft and creamy. Garnish with a small amount of chopped parsley after placing in a serving dish.

Other vegetables that go well in this soup are sweet corn, green or yellow string beans, parsley, and daikon. Whole-wheat pasta, such as elbows or shells, may also be added.

### FRIED RICE, SEOUL STYLE

4 cups cooked brown rice

$1/2$ cup tempeh (a fermented soyfood), cubed or sliced into
   thin rectangles

Dark sesame seed oil

$1/2$ cup onions, diced

$1/4$ cup mushrooms, thinly sliced

$1/4$ cup carrots, diced

Water (optional)

Tamari (naturally made soy sauce)

$1/4$ cup parsley, chopped

Place a small amount of dark sesame oil in a skillet and heat up. Add tempeh and sauté $2^1/_2$ minutes until golden brown. Add onions and mushrooms and sauté another $2^1/_2$ minutes. Add the carrots. Place the brown rice on top of the vegetables. If the rice is dry, add about $1/_8$ to $1/_4$ cup of water to steam it. Cover and turn the flame down to low. Simmer about 5 minutes or until the vegetables are tender and the rice is hot. Add a small amount of tamari and sprinkle the parsley on top of the rice. Cover and sauté another $2^1/_2$ minutes. Then remove the cover and mix the rice and vegetables together. Place in a serving bowl.

## MOZZARELLA BEAN SPROUT SANDWICH

1 cup cucumber, thinly sliced

$1/_2$ cup carrot, shredded

2 green onions, chopped

5 Tbsp. low-calorie Italian dressing

$1/_4$ cup skim mozzarella cheese, shredded

2 English muffins

$1/_4$ cup bean sprouts

Combine the cucumber, carrot, green onions and dressing together. Then sprinkle 1 Tbsp. mozzarella cheese on each half of the English muffins. Broil until melted. Spoon $1/_3$ cup of vegetable mixture on top of each half. Add 2 Tbsp. of sprouts. Yields 4 servings.

## VIETNAMESE CREAM COTTAGE CHEESE SANDWICH

$1^1/_2$ cups low-fat cottage cheese (dry curd)

$1^1/_2$ Tbsp. powdered soymilk

2 Tbsp. water

1 tsp. lemon juice

$1/_2$ cup mushrooms, chopped

1 Tbsp. onion, chopped

$1/_3$ cup carrot, chopped

$1/_4$ cup celery, chopped

1 tsp. Kyolic liquid aged garlic extract

1 tsp. natural soy sauce

Place the cottage cheese, powdered soymilk, water, and lemon juice in a Vita-Mix Total Nutrition Center (see Appendix II). Blend for 1 minute until smooth. Then scrape out the container and add the vegetables, Kyolic liquid garlic, and soy sauce.

Spread $^1/_2$ cup of this mixture on two slices of pumpernickel or rye bread to make a sandwich. Add some dark green lettuce and sliced tomatoes. This makes a creamy, crunchy sandwich.

Lunch recipes such as these satisfy hunger and provide energy, but without adding pounds. Meals like these are part of what makes the Oriental 7-day quick weight-off diet work so well.

# CHAPTER 4

# SOME FACTS YOU SHOULD KNOW ABOUT REDUCING FOODS AND FATTENING FOODS

■ ■ ■

**I**n continuing the Oriental diet for reducing without hunger, it is important that you know the truth about reducing foods and fattening foods.

This information is vitally important if you are going to embark on a reducing diet that extends beyond the seven-day period and if you want to lose from twenty to fifty pounds. In fact, this information is also important when you go on the sustaining diet to keep your weight at normal, so you will not have the perpetual struggle that plagues all dieters—a quick return of the unwanted, ugly fat!

When you have taken off the undesired weight, there will be a continual struggle all your life to keep that weight off. If you continue on the basic Oriental diet and avoid making the mistakes so many people make, you can go on to a healthier, happier life and still enjoy the foods you eat without the feelings of frustration that often beset people who think they must keep on a rigid diet the rest of their lives.

■ ■ ■

## GIRL WHO IGNORED BASIC FOOD RULES GAINED BACK LOST WEIGHT

Gladys R. weighed 150 pounds when she came to me for help. She could not stop eating fattening foods like spaghetti, mashed potatoes with gravy; creamy, rich desserts; and candies. She was given the diet regimen in Chapter 2 and it worked beautifully for her. The rice, being highly satisfying to her carbohydrate-trained taste buds, gave her great satisfaction as long as she continued eating it with the other basic diet foods. She felt satisfied, and her craving for sweets ended.

This is one of the most important things to remember in your sustaining diet: you must continue to eat some carbohydrate foods each day, but not in excess of 200 calories, otherwise the body can easily suffer from a condition known as acidosis.

Many people who eat excessive quantities of meat or other forms of proteins can also take on this condition. So Gladys was happy on her Oriental diet and kept at it until she had lost 30 pounds. Then she was at her normal weight for her height and age.

Soon, however, she began to add more carbohydrates to her diet. At noon she would sneak a malted milk. She ate one sandwich at lunch. She ate toast, butter, and marmalade for breakfast. She drank her coffee with cream and sugar, and soon she had put on 20 of the 30 pounds she had lost on her Oriental diet. Then she became really alarmed and realized that the battle against fat was a lifetime one and that she simply could not ignore basic facts about fattening and reducing foods.

It was then that I put Gladys back on the stringent Oriental diet until she was once again at her normal weight. Then I put her on a sustaining diet that included brown rice three times a week, vegetables, meat, and fruits. She was not allowed to binge on ice cream or malted milks often, and if she did, she had to diet for two extra days to catch up. Soon Gladys reported that she no longer had the craving for sweets and starches that she once had and she was holding the line at her desired weight.

■ ■ ■

## IMPORTANT TO KNOW WHEN CALORIES DO COUNT

In the battle among nutritionists regarding whether one should bother with calories or ignore them, both sides are really right, to a certain extent. In my Oriental 7-day reducing diet I do not advise you to count calories, for you can hardly eat more than 1,000 calories on the reducing soup, rice, and other limited foods given in the diet. However, you should know which foods, including meats and carbohydrates, are the highest in calories, then avoid those that are extremely high and favor those that are low. In this way, you can add variety to your reducing diet and also keep yourself on the low-calorie foods when you go on the sustaining diet.

Following are the low-calorie meats you may select from, in the Oriental system of dieting, to go with the brown rice and vegetable soup. The following calories are given for a serving of about a quarter pound of meat, or four ounces.

|  | CALORIES |
|---|---|
| Boiled beef | 211 |
| Broiled beef | 247 |
| Braised beef | 296 |
| Beef hearts | 135 |
| Beef kidneys | 225 |
| Sweetbreads | 205 |
| Lamb kidneys | 115 |
| Lamb tenderloin | 387 |
| Pork shoulder | 279 |
| Pork tenderloin | 307 |
| Ham (Yunnan Province) | 247 |

The following seafood can be utilized in place of meat for protein. It will readily be seen that seafood is usually much lower in calories than most other cuts of meat. The values cited are based on four-ounce servings.

|  | CALORIES |
|---|---|
| Prawns | 125 |
| Crab claws | 136 |
| Crabs | 167 |
| Abalone | 120 |
| Scallops | 367 |
| Carp | 116 |
| Pomfret | 248 |
| Chub's head | 108 |
| Squid | 168 |
| Perch | 220 |
| Porgy | 341 |
| Shark's fin | 148 |
| Eel | 228 |
| Salmon | 208 |
| Cod | 192 |
| Flounder | 228 |
| Sea bass | 111 |

The following poultry is frequently consumed by Orientals everywhere. These meats are relatively low in calories and can handily meet your body's protein needs during dieting. The values cited are based on four-ounce servings.

|  | CALORIES |
|---|---|
| Broiled chicken | 165 |
| Roasted chicken | 215 |
| Cold-pressed Beijing duck | 311 |
| Roasted Sichuan quail | 204 |

And while Orientals use few dairy products (except for yogurt and fermented mare's milk by the Mongolians), these foods form a vital part of any diet as low-calorie sources of valuable proteins. Values cited for the following items are based on four-ounce servings.

CALORIES

| | |
|---|---|
| Cottage cheese | 135 |
| Buttermilk | 80 |
| Skim milk | 50 |
| Evaporated milk | 185 |
| Yogurt | 85 |
| Fermented mare's milk | 72 |
| Goat milk | 96 |
| Whole cow's milk | 159 |

From these lists you may select a variety of low-calorie foods to vary any reducing plan. This may be necessary if you extend the Oriental 7-day diet to two or more weeks, and you desire to lose from twenty to fifty more pounds. Then you can eat any of the protein foods in the low-calorie lists. However, remember that these low-calorie foods can also add weight if you eat large quantities. That is why I give you the calories for an average serving of a quarter pound of meat a day. If you are trying to lose weight with the Oriental system, or any system, and you eat large quantities of even these low-calorie foods daily, exceeding 1,000 calories a day, you will hold your own, *but you will definitely not lose weight!*

Then there are the high-calorie foods that you should avoid while you are on the 7-day Oriental diet plan, and also when you are on your sustaining diet. Remember, these high-calorie foods add up more quickly on the calorie list and should be used cautiously, consuming only small portions. *They should be completely eliminated while you are on the 7-day Oriental reducing diet.*

High-calorie foods to avoid while on the 7-day Oriental diet (based on four-ounce serving):

CALORIES

| | |
|---|---|
| Frankfurters | 305 |
| Swiss steak | 400 |
| Hamburger | 390 |
| Tongue | 340 |
| Cube steak | 345 |
| Porterhouse steak | 390 |
| Rib roast | 325 |

CALORIES

| | |
|---|---|
| Chicken croquettes | 370 |
| Roasted, stuffed turkey | 490 |
| Chicken with dumplings | 540 |
| Roasted stuffed chicken | 340 |

Dairy products high in calories to avoid while dieting (calories for four ounces of weight):

CALORIES

| | |
|---|---|
| Cream | 410 |
| Butter | 920 |
| Milk (condensed, sweet) | 395 |
| Malted milk | 510 |

Calories contained by alcoholic beverages, to be avoided during 7-day Oriental diet (calories per four liquid ounces):

CALORIES

| | |
|---|---|
| Beer | 65 |
| Ale | 70 |
| Rum | 390 |
| Cognac | 240 |
| Gin | 310 |
| Champagne | 125 |
| Brandy | 240 |
| Sherry | 140 |
| Whiskey | 400 |
| Vermouth, dry | 240 |
| Vermouth, sweet | 240 |
| Vodka | 310 |
| Dry wine | 80 |
| Sweet wine | 135 |

Avoid the following foods while on your 7-day reducing plan, as they are high in calories. They can be eaten moderately after you have lost your desired amount of weight, but they should be used sparingly at all times if you wish to avoid putting the unwanted pounds back on again.

| | | |
|---|---|---|
| cakes | dressings for salads | hominy grits |
| cookies | fried eggs | fatty soups |
| candies | ice cream | sugar |
| cornstarch puddings | mayonnaise | oils of all kinds |
| jellies and marmalades | fatty meats | syrups |
| crackers | pancakes | waffles |
| sundaes, malts | sodas | |
| cornmeal | popcorn | |

■ ■ ■

## USEFUL POINTERS ON PREPARING LOW-CALORIE MEATS

In using the 7-day Oriental food plan to lose weight, you will naturally stick to the daily intake of brown rice, and the greaseless soup, that has all the reducing vegetables in it.

However, even while you are dieting, you will require some of the low-calorie meats to satisfy your body's needs for proteins. It is important that you know how to prepare these meats so as to avoid excess fats.

Of course, no meat is actually free of fat or fat calories. While on the reducing diet for the first seven days, you can have a small portion of meat each day with the rice and vegetables. However, meat should not be fried, but broiled. Meats that are fried absorb the fats and oils and increase the caloric intake nearly 100 percent.

The best way to prepare you meats, fish, chicken, or lamb, to obtain the highest benefits for a reducing regimen, is to broil them. This helps remove most of the fats, as the fat drops into the bottom of the drip pan.

You can also roast the low-calorie meats that you use in the 7-day Oriental diet plan, but be especially careful *not* to baste them. You can pour a little water over them if they should be too dry during cooking.

The Oriental diet plan suggests using more fish than other forms of protein. Substitute fish as often as possible while you are reducing, for fish is an excellent source of protein and has fewer calories than meat.

Many nutrition experts now believe that fish is a superior form of protein to meat. They ascribe the health of the Japanese people, and their high vitality and energy, to the fact that fish is high on their list of protein foods. As Japan is primarily not an agricultural country, they subsist mostly on our Oriental reducing diet products of rice, vegetables, fruits, and fish. They seldom eat red-blooded meats such as beef, and limit their intake of pork. These people are usual thin, wiry, and energetic, and they suffer less from high blood pressure, arthritis, heart trouble and other diseases that afflict the predominantly meat-eating nations of the world.

The Chinese people subsist mainly on this same diet, which I advocate for weight reduction. They eat many grains, such as rice, wheat, oats, barley, and soybeans, which are high in protein. Consequently, they stay slender and suffer from few of our modern American diseases.

Many East Indians, Tibetans, and those living in Hunza have lived to be from 110 to 135 years of age. I have investigated their diets and have found that they subsisted primarily on grains, vegetables, fruits, nuts, cheese and milk products. The Hunzas, who seem to be especially healthy and slender as well as long-lived, claim that many of their health benefits derive from the apricot, which they dry for use in the winter, and eat all year round. They claim special virtues for this golden fruit, and even believe that it gives them long life and better health. The Hunzas seldom eat red-blooded meats, subsisting entirely on a diet that would be considered inadequate in America, one of fruits, nuts, grains, vegetables, and dairy products.

■ ■ ■

## MAN I MET IN INDIA 120 YEARS OLD USED THIS DIET

I once met a man in my travels to India who was 120 years of age, and he gave me his diet, which I found was, in many ways, similar to the one we are using in our Oriental 7-day reducing diet. He was like a man of 50 or 60. He had perfect eyesight, his own teeth, a fine head of hair, and a sharp, clear mind.

I visited his home on the outskirts of Calcutta, and there he showed me his vegetable garden, where he had several different types of vegetables growing. He had two goats, from whose milk he obtained much of his protein.

This man ate whenever he felt hungry. He munched on some nuts or fruits several times a day. His main diet was a bowl of rice, goat's milk, and steamed vegetables, although he told my that he tried to eat most of his fresh vegetables raw. He had goat's cheese, occasionally an egg, and for desserts he had figs, dates, melons, and other fruits in season. The bread he served me was heavy and coarse, and he told me it was made from stone-ground wheat and barley, with goat's milk and wild honey. He told me he had not eaten meat for over 75 years, and once in a while he ate broiled fish, when some neighbor made him a special gift of fresh fish caught in a nearby stream.

This healthy Indian told me that he had tried eating red-blooded meat 75 years ago and found that it gave him such unpleasant symptoms that he stopped after a few weeks. When he stopped eating meat his condition improved at once, and he never again touched this form of protein.

He also told me that he occasionally ate lentils, and also beans. He showed me how he prepared these with onions, tomato sauce, a half cup of vegetable oil, and a little salt. He let these simmer on the stove for one or two hours, until tender, and these seemed to satisfy his protein needs. I do not recommend the bean and lentil family as foods while you are on the 7-day reducing plan, but they may occasionally be used as good sources of protein when you are on the sustaining diet, after having lost the weight you desired.

For desserts he was fond of yogurt, which he made himself from goat's milk. He put a little wild honey on this for flavor, but honey is not recommended while on your 7-day diet to lose weight, for it is a very high form of carbohydrate. It can sometimes be used for flavoring. But when you are on your sustaining diet you can use honey instead of sugar, if you wish. He also ate dates, figs, dried apricots and prunes, as well as all fruits in season. I was astonished to find that he rarely had orange juice, but he did get his Vitamin C from other foods, particularly melons, when they were in season. He also had taken a whole lemon in a glass of water, upon arising, for many years.

■ ■ ■

## HOW TO USE DAIRY PRODUCTS WHILE ON THIS REDUCING DIET

While you are on the 7-day Oriental reducing diet you can use dairy products in moderation. After you have lost the desired weight you can increase your intake of these excellent protein foods.

### *Milk*

Milk can be taken whole, either pasteurized or raw. Many nutrition experts agree that raw, unpasteurized milk is far superior to that which has been boiled. The raw milk is supervised and free of disease and contains many elements that the pasteurized milk does not contain.

Children fed on a diet of raw milk were found to be healthier and to have fewer diabetic problems than those who drank pasteurized milk. The chemistry of anything boiled, such as pasteurized milk, is changed, and the substance is no longer as valuable as a food for human beings.

Skim milk should be substituted for whole milk if you wish to avoid the fat content of whole milk during your seven-day period of reducing. When you are on your regular sustaining diet, you may take as many as two glasses of whole milk daily, if you are over twenty years of age, and at least three to four glasses if under 20 twenty (while the bones and teeth are maturing).

In considering whether you should or should not drink whole milk, realize that your body, even during periods of dieting, requires some fat to help the metabolic processes. At least two tablepoonsful of some form of fat are permissible, even while reducing. Also remember, it is not fat that makes fat in the body, but the carbohydrates, sugars, starches and certain forms of oil, such as olive oil and some animal fats.

Avoid all evaporated, canned, or condensed milk, with sugar, during this period of dieting. These are extremely high in calories and should be avoided in any weight-reducing regime.

What about cream, butter, cottage cheese, and other dairy products?

A small amount of real cream may taken in your breakfast coffee, even when reducing, as you do need some fat in your diet. Sugar can be eliminated in favor of some sugar substitute, as the sugar has calories that are converted into fat very easily. If you want to cut down on the cream in your coffee you may take a nondairy cream substitute.

Large amounts of butter should be avoided during this seven-day reducing diet, but a small amount can be used on your whole-wheat bread or toast. For salads, avoid olive oil while you are dieting because olive oil increases the caloric intake, and you can substitute corn oil, which is lower in calories and unsaturated fats. Fat that comes into the body from eating too much olive oil remains in the body longer and is most difficult to remove. This is one reason why many people in Latin countries who use excessive amounts of olive oil become very heavy as they advance in age and seldom ever lose the fat they have accumulated over years of eating olive oil.

### Cheese and Cheese Products

Most cheeses and cheese products are full of salt and other preservatives and should not be eaten in excessive amounts as part of a diet for losing weight. If less lean meat is eaten, however, some cheese may be substituted. Cottage cheese is a good substitute as it is lower in calories than other cheeses.

### Eggs

You can eat eggs in moderation while on this Oriental reducing diet, but they should not be fried; instead poach or boil them. When you fry eggs or put cream into scrambled or shirred eggs, the calorie count almost doubles.

■ ■ ■

## HOW MUCH WATER SHOULD YOUR DRINK DAILY WHILE DIETING?

Water intake should be slightly increased during the seven-day reducing period, for this reason: body fat is burned up more quickly and carried from the system if at least eight glasses of water are drunk each day. While on this 7-day reducing diet avoid drinking ice-cold water or soft drinks. The effect on the stomach is very severe when you drink ice-cold beverages. Cold water without ice is preferable.

Some reducing systems insist that you drink all the water you can daily, but this is not essential in our Oriental system of dieting. Drink when thirsty, and just before going to bed take a full glass of water. Many doctors have advised drinking water just before retiring to flush out the kidneys and to avoid the formation of kidney stones. If you awaken in the night and feel thirsty, drink one glass of water. You will find that the average person drinks far too little water, and you will have to be alert while on this reducing diet to drink sufficient amounts of water, at least 8 to 10 glasses daily, to flush out all the excess fats that your body is throwing off.

■ ■ ■
___

## SHOULD YOU BOTHER COUNTING CALORIES ON THIS DIET?

Although calories do count, you need not bother counting calories in the Oriental diet system. You can hardly eat enough soup and rice to make it worthwhile to count the calories. You will experience such a stuffed feeling on this reducing diet that you cannot possibly eat enough calories to carry you over the danger mark, about 1,200 calories.

In a weight-reducing diet such as this, calories are not important. However, I shall later give you some facts about calories and their importance in your sustaining diet. You will find that if you are a man and eat more than 1,200 calories a day, while on any reducing plan, you will not lose weight. If you are a woman and eat more than 900 calories, it will be more difficult to lose weight. You may not gain weight, and merely hold your own, but you surely will not lose weight. You do not need to actually count your calories for this short period of time. If you strictly adhere to this diet you can eat as much as you wish, until hunger is satisfied—you need not suffer from hunger. You will never gain extra pounds on this strict diet, and when you have attained your ideal weight, whether it is in one or two or three weeks, you can then be aware of calories and limit your caloric intake, as I shall instruct you in a later chapter dealing with the caloric content of various foods and what your caloric intake should be. This depends on whether you are male or female, and the nature of your work. But more about this later.

# CHAPTER 5

# VARIATIONS TO THE 7-DAY ORIENTAL REDUCING DIET

■ ■ ■

N o matter what diet system you follow there are bound to be days when the chosen diet becomes monotonous and your taste buds rebel against the sameness of the foods you eat.

Rather than abandon your Oriental 7-day diet, especially if you have gone into the second or third seven-day period and you are trying to lose from twenty to fifty more pounds, simply vary the diet, keeping to the same general plan, but with additions that will in no way keep you from losing weight but will add to the enjoyment of the new foods you will be eating.

■ ■ ■

## FIRST-DAY VARIATION DIET

### Breakfast

1 cup of orange juice, diluted with water
1 egg, boiled or poached
1 slice whole-wheat toast, with butter
Coffee or tea, artificial cream and sweetener

### Lunch

1 salmon steak, baked
Small fruit salad
1 cup of chicken-rice soup
1 medium tomato
Rice pudding

### Dinner

Baked tuna-cheese Orientale
Green beans
Small bowl of brown rice with butter
Scoop of orange or lemon sherbet
Coffee or tea, with milk and artificial sweetener

### RECIPE FOR BAKED TUNA-CHEESE ORIENTALE (FOUR SERVINGS):

Sauté 1 onion, finely chopped, in butter until golden brown. Add 2 cups skim milk until mixture is smooth and thick. Cut up 10 oz. of carrots, and add 2 cans of tuna, $1/4$ cup of whole-wheat flour, and $1/2$ cup grated cheddar cheese. Add dietetic salt to flavor; also add black pepper, a dab of mustard, and 2 small cans of tomatoes. Put this into a casserole dish and cook in a preheated oven of 375°F. Top with grated cheese, and bake for a short period of time, until the cheese has browned slightly.

You can serve this Oriental dish to guests, and they need never suspect that you are on a diet!

■ ■ ■

## SECOND-DAY VARIATION DIET

### Breakfast

Glass of orange-pineapple juice
Oatmeal with skimmed milk
2 rye or wheat thins
Coffee or tea

### Lunch

Patty of ground round, broiled
1 cup of summer squash
1 cup of asparagus
Portion of Jello (made with artificial sugar)
Coffee or tea

### Dinner

1 cup of reducing soup
5 oz. of lean leg of lamb
1 cup cooked spinach
1 small serving of brown rice
1 cup of banana whip pudding

■ ■ ■

## THIRD-DAY VARIATION DIET

### Breakfast

$1/2$ glass of apricot or prune juice
Creamed tuna on whole-wheat toast, or chipped beef on toast
   (make cream sauce with skim milk and whole-wheat flour)
Coffee or tea

**Lunch**

1 cup of consommé
1 cup of coleslaw
Tuna salad or chicken salad, with low-calorie dressing
Two pieces of zwieback toast with butter
Coffee or tea

**Dinner**

1 cup of diced cantaloupe
1 bowl of reducing soup
12 large mushrooms, broiled
1 baked potato with butter
Coffee, tea, or glass of skim milk

■ ■ ■

# FOURTH-DAY VARIATION DIET

### Breakfast

Eggs a la Shanghai (recipe below)
Glass of orange juice, diluted
Coffee, tea or skim milk

### RECIPE FOR EGGS A LA SHANGHAI (FOUR SERVINGS):

2 tsp. butter

1 small onion, finely chopped

6 chicken livers, finely chopped

$1/_2$ cup water

4 eggs

8 asparagus tips

Sauté onions in butter. Add chicken livers and brown for 5 minutes. Add water and simmer a few minutes. Scramble eggs in a separate pan that is greased with butter; cook eggs in preheated oven of 375°F for 5 minutes. Then put chicken livers over the eggs, with pieces of asparagus on top. Cook only long enough to firm eggs, and serve.

**Lunch**

Cup of reducing soup
Broiled shrimp on bed of brown rice
Salad; grapefruit slices on bed of lettuce
Coffee, tea, or skim milk

**Dinner**

Cup of reducing soup
Chinese chow mein (easy to prepare, see recipe below)

A slight variation to the monotony of lean beef, veal, chicken, and fish is sometimes necessary. In this recipe you will use a bit of diced pork, which adds a few more calories, but as they are fat calories, and your body needs some fat even when reducing, this is permissible if not overdone. (No vegetables are necessary as they are part of the chow mein.) You will need:

$1/_2$ lb. of pork, diced

3 cups of sliced Chinese cabbage

1 cup of green pepper, finely sliced

1 cup of water chestnuts

1 cup of bamboo shoots

1 cup of mushrooms

1 large onion, sliced

1 clove garlic

1 cup of bean sprouts

4 Tbsp. of soy sauce

Sauté the pork in a frying pan with little cooking oil; put all the vegetables and other ingredients into the pan and let simmer over low heat until the vegetables are cooked. Add just enough water to keep them moist while cooking.

Serve on a bed of steamed rice—either white or brown rice will do.

For dessert you may serve fresh fruit of any kind.

■ ■ ■

## FIFTH-DAY VARIATION DIET

### Breakfast

$1/_2$ glass cranberry juice
2 eggs, scrambled in butter
2 pieces of whole-wheat or protein toast
$1/_2$ tsp. jelly on toast
Coffee or tea, with cream and artificial sugar

Do not be afraid to take a little real cream for coffee occasionally, for, remember, even when reducing you need about two teaspoons of fat a day in the diet. It is generally amply furnished by the meats you eat, but occasionally you can treat yourself to some cream in your coffee without endangering the effectiveness of your reducing diet.

### Lunch

Beef-tofu hamburger (a soy sauce–flavored hamburger that combines ground beef with tofu. These small-sized burgers are tasty, soft, and pleasant to the palate, and are quite enjoyable.)

1 cup of reducing vegetable soup

Carrot-raisin salad (use shredded carrots and $1/_2$ cup of seedless raisins. Soak raisins in water until soft. Serve with a low-calorie dressing or a dressing I shall give later for salads)

Fruit, pineapple, or peach slices

Usual coffee or tea, or glass of skim milk or buttermilk

### Dinner

Sweetbreads on lean piece of ham (recipe follows)

1 lb. of lamb, beef, or sweetbreads. Boil for 10 minutes, remove from stove, drain and dry. Melt a spoonful of butter in pan, and add the sweetbreads. Add artificial salt and pepper to taste, and cook only for 2 minutes. Serve sweetbreads on a slice of pre-cooked ham, with 2 slices of protein or whole-wheat toast. Serve $1/_2$ baked potato with sour cream with this main dish.

Lemon, orange, or pineapple sherbet

■ ■ ■

## SIXTH-DAY VARIATION DIET

### Breakfast

All-wheat cereal with skim milk

1 spoonful of sugar or a little honey (not recommended for regular diet menus, but as this is a variation diet, to avoid monotony you can indulge yourself on occasion with no harm to the diet)

Fresh strawberries or other fruit

Coffee, tea, or milk

### Lunch

Salad of chopped-up vegetables in sour cream (vegetables can include cucumbers, green onions, radishes, tomatoes, and green peppers, and cut up celery stalks)

A slice of cheddar cheese

2 pieces of rye crisp or zwieback toast

Skim milk, coffee, or tea

### Dinner

Japanese beef and peppers on rice (recipe below)

Diced cooked carrots

Beef broth

Vanilla ice milk or dietetic canned fruits for dessert

Coffee, tea, or skim milk

### RECIPE FOR JAPANESE BEEF AND PEPPERS ON RICE (ONLY 200 CALORIES PER SERVING):

1 lb. ground round beef

$1/2$ tsp. minced garlic

1 tsp. salt substitute

2 beef bouillon cubes

$1/2$ tsp. of powdered ginger

8 scallions, cut in pieces
4 celery stalks, cut in $^1/_2$-inch pieces
4 medium green peppers, cut into strips
2 Tbsp. of cornstarch
1 Tbsp. of soy sauce
$^1/_2$ cup water
2 Tbsp. of oil

Shape the ground beef into small patties. Brown them in oil and the minced garlic. Put in the beef bouillon cubes, ginger, salt and pepper; cover with hot water and simmer for 15 minutes. Then add the vegetables and cook until vegetables are tender. Put the cornstarch, soy sauce, and water together, and mix thoroughly, then add to the other ingredients in the skillet and cover it, cooking it about 10 more minutes, or until vegetables are tender.

■ ■ ■

## SEVENTH-DAY VARIATION DIET

### Breakfast

$^1/_2$ honeydew melon
$^1/_2$ cup yogurt
1 slice whole-wheat or rye bread toasted
Coffee or tea

### Lunch

1 cup of consommé
2 celery stalks and radishes
Calf's liver, broiled
4 wheat thins
Coffee or tea

### Dinner

1 glass tomato juice
Bass, or other fish, broiled or baked only
$^1/_2$ cup of brown rice with butter over it
Fresh fruit, or one-half canned peach
Coffee or tea

Between meals, while on this variation diet, you can eat a bowl of the reducing soup whenever you feel hungry. These variation diets can also be interspersed with the regular reducing diets given in the second chapter, to add variety and to help sustain you if you have to go beyond the seven-day period of dieting.

Later I shall give many other menus that will add variety to your regular meals when you go on the sustaining diet to maintain your normal weight.

■ ■ ■

## OTHER POINTERS TO FOLLOW DURING THE 7-DAY DIET

1. Avoid table salt, which is sodium chloride, using a salt substitute instead. If you eat in restaurants, the food will already be salted, so avoid putting extra salt on the food.

   Your body can absorb only three hundred grains of salt a day, and each shake of the salt-cellar gives about a thousand grains. The excess salt is stored in the body tissues with large quantities of liquids. This is why the first two or three days of fasting and dieting generally make you lose three or four pounds of weight—most of it is water that has been held in solution in the tissues by the salt you have ingested for years.

2. Avoid reducing pills or other drugs while you are on this diet (exceptions: those who have diabetes or other illnesses that require a doctor's care). Check with your doctor before you embark on any reducing diet, and occasionally while on the diet, to be sure you are maintaining your usual level of energy and good health.

3. I always suggest that you take a good vitamin pill that contains all the essential vitamins, minerals, and other elements that have been judged as being essential to good health. However, avoid overdoing, as it has been found by medical research that most people overdo in taking vitamins without a doctor's advice, and more harm can be done than good. Later we shall discuss vitamins in further detail.

4. If you feel weak after a day or two of this reducing diet and you want a quick pickup, do not mistakenly eat sugar, candy, or honey, thinking your body needs sugar for quick energy. Your body needs the sugar that comes from natural fruits or fruit juices. But rather than drink too much fruit juice while on this diet, eat the natural oranges and other fruits, whenever possible. The reason for this is simple: the juices are quickly absorbed into your system and require no digestion, whereas the whole fruits, with their pulp, require a longer time to digest and make the stomach work. If you eat an apple when hungry, or stewed apples, or baked apples without sugar, your body is given quick energy without adding to the fat problem.

5. Avoid eating anything just before retiring at night. The body requires very few calories while you sleep, and these are adequately furnished by your normal evening meal.

   If you do feel hungry at night or during the night, drink a glass of skim milk or eat some kind of fruit, such as melon, apples, two or three prunes, dried apricots, or other fruits in season. You can also nibble on a piece of cheese to appease your appetite.

# CHAPTER 6

# WHAT YOU SHOULD KNOW ABOUT CALORIES, VITAMINS, AND FOODS TO NEVER AGAIN PUT ON WEIGHT

■ ■ ■

The biggest problem facing any dieter is the fact that he can, and often does, take off weight following this Oriental 7-day system of dieting, but within a few weeks' time, through carelessness or not knowing food values, he puts the weight back on again.

It is disheartening to lose weight and then see the scales registering those lost pounds in a few weeks' time. This is why it is vitally important that you know the truth about calories, vitamins, minerals, and foods in general, so that you can go on a sustaining diet that will be nutritious and at the same time keep the unwanted pounds off.

Although you do not need to count calories during the 7-day quick weight-off diet given in this book, it is important that you know something about calories so you can avoid overloading the body with unneeded calories in the future. It must always be remembered that even if you ate nothing but meat, but overate of it, thus absorbing more calories than the body can use, the extra calories would be stored by the body as fat. Of course, carbohydrates, starches, and sugars are converted into fat much quicker than lean meat is, and these should be lowered drastically on any sustaining diet to keep your body at normal weight.

A calorie is the standard unit for measuring food energy. The calorie used in nutrition is the kilocalorie (kcal) or large calorie (Cal). This unit is one thousand times larger than the small calorie (cal) used in chemistry and physics. The word *calorie*, which is often used to describe the potential energy of food, is a unit of measure of heat (not nutritional value). The following table (courtesy of the National Academy of Science and the National Research Council in Washington, D.C.) gives the recommended caloric intake per day for men and women of different ages.

|  | *Age* | *Energy (kcal)* |
|---|---|---|
| Males | 19–22 | 3,000 |
|  | 23–50 | 2,700 |
|  | 51+ | 2,400 |
| Females | 19–22 | 2,100 |
|  | 23–50 | 2,000 |
|  | 51+ | 1,800 |
| Pregnant |  | +300 |
| Lactating |  | +500 |

The recommended calories per day for the average person, released recently by scientific sources are as follows: 2,400 to 3,000 calories for men, depending on their weight, age, and height. The recommended number of calories per day for the average woman is between 1,800 and 2,100 calories.

Men who do heavy labor require up to 3,500 calories a day to keep them in good condition. If they consume 4,000 or more calories a day they are going to put on excess weight. In the category of heavy labor I include people who use their muscles in lifting or moving heavy objects, like furniture, machinery, or packing crates filled with heavy objects. Truck drivers who do not lift heavy loads but merely drive their trucks would hardly be classified as heavy laborers. They actually have sedentary jobs and require no more than 2,500 calories per day. This is one reason why most truck drivers you see on the road weigh from twenty-five to eighty pounds too much. They stop at roadside cafes to eat mostly carbohydrate foods such as sandwiches, pies, cakes, ice cream, coffee and doughnuts, and other starches. All those fat calories are stored as fat.

Cutting out at least 50 percent of the carbohydrates you would normally eat on the sustaining diet will help you keep the body at its normal weight. This, of course, means that you should balance the diet with adequate amounts of proteins, vegetables, and fruits.

Each day part of the calorie content should be of a high-protein nature. It is estimated that men require at least 350 protein calories a day and that women require at least 290 protein calories. No adequate research has ever been made of carbohydrate requirements per day. If you play safe by keeping on a very low carbohydrate diet, you will get immediate results in your program for losing weight. This is why the Oriental 7-day diet works miracles—it furnishes the body with vegetables and meat protein, allowing for a small intake of carbohydrates in the brown rice, with plenty of fats and sugars for energy, without danger of storing the excess sugar as fat.

The basic reason why people are overweight is that their bodies do not burn up carbohydrates easily, storing these carbohydrates as fat instead. This is one good reason for reducing the intake of carbohydrates and substituting meat, vegetables, and natural fruits for a maintenance diet that will be nutritious and yet keep off future weight.

■ ■ ■

## THE NEED FOR VITAMINS AND MINERALS

One of the main worries of many people who undertake the 7-day Oriental diet is whether they will obtain sufficient vitamins and minerals while on the diet. They often ask: are vitamins necessary as a daily supplement to the reducing diet and afterward on the sustaining diet?

It has been scientifically established that the body requires certain vitamins and minerals, which could normally be supplied by food, if we all ate correctly. But this is difficult to do, and it is recommended by most doctors and nutritionists that supplementary vitamins be taken while on reducing diets and then on sustaining diets. Here is the logical reason for this: during the many years of reaping crops without enriching the soil, we have witnessed a gradual deterioration of the soil, especially in this country. Although farmers are now trying to restore the balance with fertilizers, many people feel that artificial fertilizers do more harm than good. The foods are then further processed and devitalized in our modern manufacturing plants, and many people believe that the foods are robbed of their nutritive elements and that most of the vitamins and minerals are destroyed. Fruits, which normally are nourishing if allowed to ripen on the trees, are picked while unripe and allowed to ripen in the markets. All these practices tend to destroy nature's balance and cause many of our processed foods to lack the vitamins and minerals they should have.

### The Value of Vitamins and Minerals

For many years scientists attempted to prove the need for vitamins and minerals in the human diet. They experimented at first with rats and found that when deprived of certain elements in their daily diets the rats suffered from every known complaint from arthritis to sterility. But people said, "Rats are not human beings, and they do not react in the same way to dietary deficiencies."

It was then that scientists began to experiment with vitamin therapy on human beings, and they soon found out that what applied to the animals in their laboratory experiments also applied to human beings.

When vitamins were restricted it was found that people became highly nervous and neurotic. They tired easily and had no resistance to disease, catching colds quickly, especially when deprived of the important vitamin C in their diets. Calcium deficiencies soon produced difficulties in metabolism and nutrition, as well as tooth and bone formation.

Perhaps the greatest proof of the need for certain vitamins and elements in the diet is that furnished by history. A naval doctor observed that the crews of British ships suffered from scurvy on long ocean voyages when they were denied fresh vegetables and fruits. He tried giving the sick men fresh lemons and the signs of scurvy completely disappeared.

Another scientist noted that when laboratory rats were given a diet of protein and carbohydrates, and nothing else, they became sick. He added whole milk to their diets, and the rats became healthy once again. The scientists concluded then by scientists that to be healthy one required a diet made up of proteins and carbohydrates and certain other unknown elements. It was a Polish chemist named Casimir Funk who discovered what these other unknown elements were, and he called them vitamins.

Scientists estimate that thirteen vitamins are essential to good health. As many as fifty vitamins have been isolated in recent years, but not all of them are considered essential to maintaining good health. Some scientists claim that at least twenty-five of these known vitamins are important to the proper functioning of the body.

We shall consider a few of the vitamins that have been proved essential to human nutrition. You may consult your doctor to see if you need special vitamin therapy, or if you can take one capsule a day, which contains most of the vitamins and minerals thought necessary for human nutrition. She will recommend the particular brand that she feels is best for your special needs.

### Vitamin A

This is the vitally important vitamin that helps protect your body against infections. It is also thought that when the body does not have sufficient vitamin A there may be deficiencies in fertilization and difficulties in the growth of the embryo in the mother's womb. This often causes childbirth disturbances.

Vitamin A is also thought to be important to full bone formation. A lack of this vitamin can also affect digestion adversely, and sometimes cause respiratory disturbances. Insufficient quantities are also thought to cause premature aging, and many scientists believe sufficient quantities of vitamin A add extra years to life.

How can you obtain vitamin A from natural foods? You can find this important vitamin in many green vegetables, including turnip greens, broccoli, squash, dandelions, collards, and mustard greens.

Vitamin A is also found in carrots, apricots, cantaloupes, and other yellow fruits and vegetables. Fish liver oils, liver, eggs, cream, and butter are also heavy in vitamin A. It is estimated by scientists that the human body puts fat on more rapidly when it is deprived of vitamin A, and they recommend at least 10,000 units a day.

### Vitamin B₁ (Thiamine)

The B vitamins are all essential to good health and balanced nutrition. Vitamin $B_1$, which contains thiamine, seems to be necessary for the proper functioning of the heart muscle and the body muscles as well as the entire nervous system. It also regulates the action of the adrenal glands when a person is threatened.

Modern research on this important vitamin shows that a lack of it causes a person to lose his sexual desires. The symptoms of a lack of vitamin $B_1$ are irritability, quick temper, nervousness, fatigue, constipation, indigestion, distended abdomen, a loss of desire for food, and, very often, dry hair.

Vitamin $B_1$ has been called the vitality vitamin by some, and it can be obtained in its natural form in such foods as soybeans, brown rice, wheat germ, brewer's yeast, beef kidneys, beef heart, oysters, some pork products, and eggs. As this vitamin is easily destroyed by heat, one should avoid overcooking and be sure to get it in such foods as yeast, wheat germ, and oysters eaten on the half shell.

### Vitamin B₂ (Riboflavin)

When this vitamin is missing in the diet it can affect the eyes, often causing burning, itching, and a bloodshot condition. When there is a lack of this important vitamin the body seems to age faster and has less resistance to fatigue. Very often its lack shows in skin disorders, such as dandruff and eczema. Scientists noted that lack of this vitamin can also cause depression, loss of hair, and a general diminished vitality that affects sexual potency.

This vitamin can be obtained from the following foods: milk, eggs, cheese, wheat germ, brewer's yeast, liver, green vegetables, peas, lima beans, yogurt, and whole-wheat cereals, and flour. If you eat plenty of yeast and liver you will obtain adequate amounts of riboflavin in your diet.

## Vitamin $B_6$ (Pyridoxine)

Until recently this little-known vitamin was considered nonessential to human nutrition. Recent research shows that pyridoxine is important for the metabolism of proteins and helps form antibodies that fight germ infections and aid in healing. It has also been found to have a sedative effect on the nerves and improves muscle tone. It is being widely used today in the treatment of muscular dystrophy and multiple sclerosis, as well as for other disorders affecting the nerves and muscles.

This vitamin is to be found in whole-wheat foods, bran, and cereals, as well as in most meats. Liver is very high in this vitamin, and so are fresh, green, leafy vegetables.

## Niacin (Vitamin B)

Niacin is part of the entire B complex and is essential for oxidizing carbohydrates and building enzymes that give mental well-being, as well as healthy skin. Niacin is vitally important to the operation of the human brain and the nervous system. When it is lacking in the human diet it often leads to nervous disorders ranging from simple nervousness to insanity. It can also contribute to hair growth and healthy hair through its effect on the blood's circulation to the scalp.

Niacin can be found in natural foods such as liver, lean meats, fish, poultry, bran, and yeast. It also exists in the leafy green vegetables.

## Vitamin $B_{12}$

Since 1948, when this vitamin was first isolated, it was recommended for the treatment of pernicious anemia. Now it has been found that this vitamin is essential for the proper functioning of the body's metabolism. Sufficient quantities of vitamin $B_{12}$ in the human diet result in mental alertness and physical vigor. It has also been found essential in normal functioning of bone marrow, as it contains an essential element, cobalt. This vitamin has been found to stimulate growth in retarded children. When this essential vitamin is lacking in the diet, disturbances in the nervous system arise, and one is deprived of the true enjoyment that comes from sexual relations. It has also been found necessary for avoiding pernicious anemia.

This vitally important vitamin is not to be found in vegetables. It is found only in meat, especially liver, and milk. The organ meats are especially good sources. It can also be found in fish, eggs, and milk products such as cottage cheese and yogurt.

### Other B Vitamins

Most vitamin tablets on the market today contain other members of the B-vitamin family, and, some consider these members essential to human nutrition. Following is a brief description of the these vitamins in the B complex, and what is known about their effects on human nutrition.

PANTOTHENIC ACID. This form of the B-complex vitamin affects the absorption of carbohydrates and the body's metabolism. It also has a strong effect on the functioning of the adrenal glands, which secrete the hormone known as adrenaline. Pantothenic acid is also thought to be important for mental health, as it reacts favorably on the nervous system and when the mind and body are under stress conditions. Some research has been done in the field of gray hair and pantothenic acid, and it is claimed that lack of this B vitamin in the diet often leads to premature graying of the hair.

Pantothenic acid is found in liver, kidney, heart, yeast, egg yolk, black molasses, rice bran and wheat bran, peas, and peanuts.

CHOLINE. This member of the B-complex family is said to be important in the absorption of fats and also prevents fatty degeneration of the liver. It is also said to control the transmission of nerve impulses from the brain to the body's muscles and organs. Choline is to be found in its natural state in beef heart, egg yolk, legumes, whole-grain cereals, and green vegetables.

INOSITOL. This B-complex vitamin seems to join in with choline to help the body absorb fatty foods, and also to protect the liver. It has also been found important in helping the stomach pass food through the intestines, a process known as peristalsis. It is to be found in organ meats, most meats, soybeans, citrus fruits, and cereal brans.

FOLIC ACID. This is the B-complex vitamin that is thought by scientists to be important to the building of normal red blood cells, and it also helps fight anemia. It gives the body the ability to fight the stressful conditions produced by modern living and helps build the antibodies that fight germ invasion of the body. It can be found in such foods as liver, organ meats, kidneys, yeast, whole wheat, veal, beef, and salmon, and to some extent in green leafy vegetables.

BIOTIN. This B-complex vitamin is important to the proper functioning of the enzymes in the body fluids and also assists the respiratory system. It can be obtained in most meats, in liver and kidneys, in egg yolk, yeast, vegetables, milk, nuts, grains, and molasses.

You can use wheat and corn germ as a daily food supplement to assure that you are getting many of the important B vitamins in your diet. Use wheat germ or corn germ over your salads and use wheat germ instead of bread crumbs to coat fish, veal, or other meats when you want to bake or fry them.

Add a tablespoon of food yeast to your stews, gravies, and even tomato juice.

Eat at least two glasses of yogurt a day while on your sustaining diet, and also use yogurt instead of mayonnaise or sour cream to make your salad dressings.

Try to eat broiled liver at least twice a week, and remember, beef liver is just as good as calf's liver, and less expensive.

### Vitamin C

There has been a great deal of controversy regarding vitamin C in relation to building the body's immunity to colds and infections. However, scientists think it has other important functions in the human body and is essential in the diet.

Vitamin C is involved in building resistance to infections, and also the body's healing. It helps maintain the cartilage, bones, and teeth in good condition. It also helps support the body's network of small blood vessels, veins, and capillaries in good condition, and causes them to function more efficiently.

Vitamin C is not stored in the body and has to be supplied daily through the diet or through other sources.

Vitamin C is to be found abundantly in all citrus fruits, oranges, lemons, grapefruit, tomatoes, limes, raspberries, black currants, raw cabbage, green peppers, cauliflower, kale, parsley, watercress, broccoli, spinach, and new potatoes.

### Vitamin D

This vitamin is thought to be essential for the formation of good bones and teeth, and also for calm nerves and to assist the body to achieve normal growth. It also helps the metabolism of phosphorus and calcium.

Vitamin D is called the "sunshine vitamin" because it is contained in abundance in the sun's rays, and those who sunbathe a good deal absorb this important vitamin. It can also be obtained in capsules of fish liver oils. Only a few foods contain this important vitamin: irradiated yeast, eggs, milk, and such fish as tuna, salmon, sardines, and mackerel.

### Vitamin E

This vitamin is considered essential to the normal functioning of the cardiovascular system. It is often called the sex vitamin and is thought to be important in maintaining sexual potency as well as for the proper functioning of the reproductive glands. A lack of vitamin E in animals has been found to lead to a degeneration of the testicles and sterility. Now many doctors are treating impotency in men and frigidity in women with diets rich in vitamin E. It is also thought important for the control of unpleasant symptoms in menopause, and for eliminating hot flashes, excessive menstrual flow, and backache. When taken with vitamin A, it is also found to help protect against liver disorders, dry skin, and persistent headaches, and it is said to be an aid in hair and skin beauty.

Vitamin E is to be found in wheat germ oil, corn germ and oil, soy oil, muscular meats, nuts, eggs, legumes, and green leafy vegetables.

### Vitamin F

This vitamin is a key factor in the absorption of other vitamins, and it is said to distribute calcium; it is also a contributing factor to the maintenance of good health and growth. When this vitamin is lacking it is found that a person can have a tendency to arteriosclerosis. It helps the body resist disease and assists the body in maintaining its proper cholesterol level. This vitamin is found in grain and vegetable oils, wheat germ, safflower, peanut, soybean, and sunflower oils. Using these oils in salads and cooking will supply the body's normal needs of vitamin F.

### Vitamin K

Scientists have recently reported that vitamin K is important to the normal clotting of the blood and to the prevention of hemorrhage. In Japan recently, scientists claimed that vitamin K is vitally important in human longevity. This vitamin is to be found in spinach, kale, cabbage, tomatoes, soybeans, liver, and vegetable oils. It is also to be found in egg yolk and alfalfa.

### Vitamin P

Also known as the bioflavenoids. The components of the bioflavenoids are citrin, hesperidin, rutin, flavones, and flavonals. This vitamin is essential to the normal health of the capillary system and is thought to be important to sexual arousal. It has another vital function—cell feeding and the removal of waste products from the body. It also gives protection against many diseases and the malfunctioning of many of the body's vital processes. It is to be found in plums, prunes, grapes, spinach, parsley, green peppers, citrus fruits, lettuce, cabbage, watercress, apples, and carrots. Paprika is also a good source of this vitamin.

■ ■ ■

## THE IMPORTANCE OF MINERALS IN ANY DIET

Most people know a great deal about the importance of vitamins in the diet, but little about minerals. These are now considered important in the diet, for minerals and vitamins work together. There are at least sixteen minerals in our foods, but we will consider only eight of the most important ones. Again, these are generally included with vitamins, but they can also be obtained from natural foods.

### Calcium

Calcium is well known as the builder of bones and teeth and for the maintenance of the body's skeletal structure. Vitamin D is important in conjunction with calcium for it helps the body absorb calcium from the stomach and digestive tract and helps the body utilize it. It has also been found that calcium is essential to a balanced, calm nervous system.

Calcium needs to be replenished often, for if the body lacks this vital mineral, it borrows it from the bones.

Calcium is found plentifully in the following foods: milk, most cheeses, blackstrap molasses, buttermilk, lemons, oranges, powdered skim milk, yogurt, leafy vegetables, cottage cheese, seafood, whole grains, egg yolk, and poultry.

### Iron

Iron is essential in the diet because it helps the blood carry oxygen throughout the body and also helps eliminate carbon dioxide from the body's cells.

Iron is essential for avoiding anemia and maintaining the bloodstream in good health. It also contributes to quicker thinking and gives the body more vital energy.

Foods that are rich in iron are liver, yeast, blackstrap molasses, barley, wheat germ, whole wheat, dried apricots, and peaches, navy and kidney beans, soybeans, lean meats, bran, eggs, lentils, oysters, prunes, and raisins.

### Iodine

Iodine is thought important for the normal functioning of the thyroid gland and to help the body's metabolism. When people are easily fatigued and feel a letdown around midday, it is usually because they lack this vital mineral in their diets. When a severe case of iodine deficiency exists it can even lead to the formation of a goiter. Iodine can be found in seafood, principally shrimp, lobster, oysters, sea greens, and iodized salt.

### Phosphorus

It is thought that phosphorus works like calcium in the body, and is closely associated with it in sustaining the fluid content of the brain. It also helps reinforce the nerves and muscles. Phosphorus aids the glands in their proper secretions and assists the muscles in their contractions. It is to be found in the following foods: meats, fish, eggs, cheese, poultry, whole wheat, and soybeans.

### Manganese

The first place that an absence of this vital mineral is noticed is in a loss of interest in sex. When manganese is lacking in the diet it can impair normal reproductive functions and often lessens the maternal instinct in women. This vital mineral activates the enzymes and works with calcium and phosphorus. It is to be found in whole grains, cereals, and green vegetables.

### Copper

This mineral helps one avoid anemia, for it works in conjunction with iron. It also plays a part in pigment formation, and a deficiency in copper can sometimes lead to prematurely gray hair. Copper is to be found in the same foods that are rich in iron, and also in oatmeal and huckleberries.

### Sodium

Sodium is essential for the absorption of all the other minerals. Sodium is plentiful in celery, green string beans, and kelp or sea salt.

*Potassium*

This mineral is called nerve food, for it helps the nerves, assists the heart and muscles, and is generally important in avoiding indigestion, constipation, insomnia, nervousness, and irritability. Potassium is found in green leafy vegetables, carrots, cucumbers, kelp, cranberries, tomatoes, apple cider vinegar, blackstrap molasses, honey, and many fruits.

With this knowledge to fortify you, you can make your own decision whether you need vitamin-and-mineral supplements in your reducing or maintenance diet. You may feel that you obtain sufficient amounts in your normal diet of both vitamins and minerals. If there is any doubt or you have some special condition that gives you problems, be sure to consult your family physician for more specific guidance.

# CHAPTER 7

# EXCITING NEW DISHES TO SUPPLEMENT THE ORIENTAL QUICK WEIGHT-LOSS PLAN

O ne of the most difficult things for a dieter to face is the deadly monotony of any reducing diet. However, using our basic diet for reducing without hunger, we can add exciting new dishes that give nourishing meals as well as exciting the taste buds.

These dishes, in conjunction with the basic Oriental diet plan, will add variety to your reducing menus, without adding weight.

Fish is one of the best sources of protein in any reducing diet. A wide variety of this delicious protein food is available, and it may be prepared in many tasty dishes that can add variety to your reducing-without-hunger diet.

A delicious reducing salad may be prepared for guests, who will never suspect you are on a diet, as follows:

Shanghai tuna and shrimp salad to be served on a bed of cold
lettuce

Two or three cans of white meat chunk tuna

One pound of cooked shrimps

One small chopped onion

Bits of green pepper or red pepper to add color, finely chopped

Add dried tarragon, or a touch of tarragon vinegar to the following reducing mayonnaise.

### REDUCING MAYONNAISE

2 Tbsp. of tarragon vinegar or lemon juice

1 egg yolk

1 tsp. honey

$1/2$ tsp. salt or substitute

1 tsp. dry mustard

$1/2$ tsp. ginger

Touch of black pepper

$1/4$ tsp. paprika

$1/4$ tsp. basil

1 cup soy oil

Blend these ingredients in a blender, except the oil and half the
vinegar, which should be added slowly while blending the other
ingredients. Add the oil slowly, and also the reserved vinegar,
until the mixture begins to thicken and then add all the oil.

Mix the ingredients of the salad with enough homemade mayonnaise to make it tasty, and serve on a bed of cold lettuce.

### LOBSTER CANTONESE

You can use frozen lobster tails for this delicious protein substitute in your reducing diet or in the sustaining diet, as it nour-
ishes without adding weight.

6 rock lobster tails (remove the undershell)

$3/4$ cup of salad oil

Juice of one lemon

$3/4$ tsp. salt or salt substitute

2 large garlic cloves, minced

$1/8$ tsp. of black pepper

Several sprigs of parsley

Mix the ingredients in a bowl and marinate the lobster tails in this mixture for about 1 hour. Then broil the tails in a hot oven, shell side up. Serve with lemon and butter sauce.

### INDONESE FILLETS OF FISH IN WINE SAUCE

1 lb. fish fillets

1 onion, finely chopped

1 Tbsp. butter

1 clove garlic, minced

1 medium can of tomatoes

$1/2$ cup of white wine

1 Tbsp. chopped parsley

$1/4$ tsp. oregano

2 Tbsp. cream

Salt and pepper to taste

First, cut fillets in half. Brown the onion and garlic in a pan with butter. Cover the fish with tomatoes, wine, and parsley. After bringing to a boil, cover and simmer over low fire for about 20 minutes. Then add the oregano and cream, stirring it until it is smooth. Garnish with parsley and serve.

### SINGAPORE PORK BAKED OVER CHARCOAL

2 lbs. lean pork (to serve about 6 guests)

1 cup of salted almonds

2 cloves garlic, minced

2 Tbsp. ground coriander seeds

Crushed red pepper

3 medium-sized onions, finely chopped

3 Tbsp. lemon juice

2 Tbsp. brown sugar

$^1/_4$ cup soy sauce

$^1/_2$ cup melted butter

$^1/_2$ cup chicken bouillon

Salt and pepper to taste

(to be served on a bed of cooked brown rice)

Cut the pork into cubes about 1 inch square. (Trim off all the fat.) Put all the ingredients except the chicken bouillon and butter into a blender and make a puree of it. Boil this and then add the melted butter and bouillon. Let this mixture cool, and then pour over the chunks of pork and let stand two hours. Put the meat on iron skewers and broil over charcoal fire. Use the left-over sauce to baste occasionally while cooking and then serve on a bed of brown rice, with the balance of the sauce.

### CURRY OF LOBSTER INDIENNE

This delicious dish may often be substituted for the other forms of meat to add variety in your seven-day diet. Or if you continue the reducing diet for a two- or three-week period, it is important that you use these variations to your regular diet plan or you will suffer from the usual monotony that afflicts most dieters and makes them give up before achieving their desired weight loss.

| | |
|---|---|
| 3 or 4 lbs. parboiled lobster | 1 Tbsp. coriander |
| 2 sliced tomatoes | Pinch of salt |
| 2 sliced onions | 1 tsp. sugar |
| pinch of cinnamon | 1 Tbsp. lemon juice |
| Cumin | 2 cloves garlic, minced |
| Cloves | 4 cups of skim milk |
| Chili powder | 1 cucumber, thinly sliced |
| 6 Tbsp. butter | 1 Tbsp. turmeric |

Fry the sliced onions with the cloves, cumin, chili, coriander, cinnamon, turmeric, and tomatoes in 3 tbs. of butter. Then add the sugar, salt, lemon juice, and milk to the mixture. Simmer on low heat for 15 minutes. Then add the other 3 Tbsp. of butter in another pan and slightly fry the garlic in it. Add the lobster and coat it well with butter. Cook for only 5 or 6 minutes, then add the milk and spices. Cook until the liquid has been reduced by almost one third. Keep pan covered while cooking. Then add thinly sliced cucumbers to the lobster and cook for an additional 10 minutes. It may be served on a bed of cooked brown rice.

### ORIENTAL GREEN PEPPERS AND BEAN SPROUTS

To add variety to your lunches while reducing, you can serve this delicious dish for guests who need never know you are on a reducing diet. This may be served as the vegetable dish with a tuna salad or some other form of broiled fish.

2 cups of bean sprouts (precook 10 minutes and drain.)

1 medium green pepper cut in rings

2 tsp. sherry extract

2 tsp. soy sauce

1 tsp. vinegar

Cook together the bean sprouts, green peppers, sherry extract, and soy sauce over moderate heat for about 15 minutes. Then add salt and vinegar and serve as a side dish with either a fish or lean meat meal.

### JAPANESE FISH FILLETS AND GREEN PEAS

This delicious fish dish can be served for either lunch or dinner. In addition, to add filler, you may take a bowl of brown rice or another vegetable from our reducing list of vegetables, such as asparagus, spinach, cabbage, or celery.

2 lb. of fish fillets, cut up in 2- × 3-inch pieces

1 cup of chicken bouillon

1 clove garlic, minced

5 oz. sliced scallions

2 Tbsp. minced ginger root or $^1/_4$ tsp. ground ginger

1 tsp. salt

1 cup  peas

1 tsp. soy sauce

1 tsp. artificial sweetener, or enough to equal 1 tsp. sugar

In a Teflon pan cook together the chicken bouillon and the ginger root until it comes to a boil. Then add scallions, garlic, and fish chunks, cooking lightly for about 5 minutes. When the fish flakes easily, add peas, soy sauce, sugar, and salt. Cook only about 5 minutes, then serve. Makes about 4 servings.

### VEAL ORIENTALE

Veal is an excellent form of meat for you while you are on this Oriental reducing diet. It can be combined with the vegetables in our reducing list and can also be served with a bowl of rice. This dish is easy to prepare and adds variety for the taste buds.

2 pieces of boneless veal cut into 1-inch cubes

4 tsp. sherry extract

$^1/_2$ cup water

$^1/_4$ cup soy sauce

2 Tbsp. salt or substitute

2 slices of ginger root, or a pinch of ground ginger

1 tsp. artificial sweetener

Garnish with watercress

In a saucepan brown the veal thoroughly over low fire. Add the sherry and water, soy sauce, salt, and ginger. Mix thoroughly, and then add the browned veal. Reduce heat after bringing to a boil, and cook over low heat for 1 hour, covered. Then add the sweetener, and cook until tender, which should be about $^1/_2$ hour longer. Serve on a bed of brown rice, with watercress garnish.

### HONG KONG PORK AND VEGETABLES

3 medium green peppers, cut in strips

2 lb. lean pork, thinly sliced

1 cup of sliced mushrooms

$1/8$ tsp. black pepper

$1/8$ tsp. ground ginger

$1/8$ tsp. nutmeg

$1/8$ tsp. salt

1 Tbsp. soy sauce

1 cup onion bouillon or onion soup

$1/2$ cup celery, chopped

2 pimentos, cut into pieces (for garnish)

2 cups of brown rice (to be served as side dish)

Combine the onions, green peppers, mushrooms, celery, salt, pepper, ginger, onion bouillon, nutmeg, sherry extract, and soy sauce. Cover over and cook on low fire for 10 minutes. By this time the onions and celery should be tender but not overcooked.

Now add the pork and pimentos, and mix well, cooking for an additional four or five minutes.

Serve with brown rice as a side dish.

### SHRIMP WITH BAMBOO SHOOTS

Another excellent Oriental diet dish consists of celestial shrimp and bamboo shoots. You may obtain these in most markets in cans. This can be served as the main dinner dish with a generous helping of brown rice with soy sauce. You will need:

2 lb. of cooked shrimp

1 Tbsp. soy sauce

4 tsp. sherry extract

1 tsp. artificial sugar

8 oz. scallions, cut up

$1/2$ tsp. black pepper

1 can bamboo shoots

Combine the soy sauce, sherry extract, and artificial sweetener in a pan, with black pepper. In another pan put the shrimp, bamboo shoots, and scallions. Then pour the sauce over the shrimp and cook over low heat for about 5 or 6 minutes. Serve with a dish of brown rice on the side.

### INDONESE BARBECUED CHICKEN

2 lb. of boned chicken (four servings)

$^1/_2$ tsp. cumin

$^1/_2$ tsp. minced garlic

6 oz. water

$^3/_4$ tsp. vinegar

Salt to taste

Cut the chicken into pieces of about 2 inches square and place them on skewers. Dip the chicken in the sauce made of the above ingredients, and cook for about 20 minutes over an open fire. Make the following sauce to serve with the chicken.

$^1/_2$ cup chicken bouillon

5 Tbsp. peanut butter

1 tsp. sugar substitute

1 clove garlic, minced

1 tsp. soy sauce

Dash of paprika

4 oz. milk

1 bay leaf

Mix these sauce ingredients thoroughly and cook slightly, until they are blended. Then serve this sauce hot over the chicken.

■ ■ ■

## PROPOSED ONE-DAY MENU WITH JAPANESE DISHES FOR DIETERS SEEKING MORE VARIETY

In 1991, Wakunaga of America and its parent company, Wakunaga Pharmaceutical Company of Hiroshima, arranged a two-week, all-expenses-paid trip to Japan for about two dozen people from several different countries. There were people representing the media, medicine, science, and business. Earl Mindell, popular nutrition writer, and I were two of those in this group.

Our visit to "the Land of the Rising Sun" allowed us to see many aspects of Japanese life in an unhurried, orderly fashion. We had the opportunity to see how Kyolic garlic (the world's leading and most respected brand of garlic) was made. We followed its progress from rows of tiny seedlings in a field to its aging phase in gigantic tanks, all the way to its finished form in hundreds of thousands of bottles rolling off the plant assembly line.

Our gracious hosts afforded us ample time to inspect Japanese cuisine and investigate other unique aspects of this rather impressive lifestyle. Through the assistance of capable translators, the material presented here was obtained from different chefs I interviewed while there.

Dieting is hard enough to begin with. But when the dieter is faced with a limited choice of foods, the experience can eventually become more burdensome that it really should. I asked Dr. Mindell how he and his wife were able to keep their own weight in reasonable check. His reply surprised me and was the inspiration for scrutinizing Japanese food preferences more carefully. He said, "My wife and I discovered some years ago that by eating many of the things the Japanese like, it helped to hold our weights down. We've always had our fair share of the 'battle of the bulge,' but once we switched to this type of Oriental cuisine, our struggles weren't as severe. It's been a great diet for us to keep our bodies in good physical shape without denying ourselves many of the things {mostly seafood) we like to eat."

The sample menu of dishes offered for a three-meal day is fairly typical for the average Japanese diet. The recipes follow; most of the ingredients called for are readily obtainable in any Japanese and Oriental food market in larger cities. Hopefully, this short introduction to some exciting dishes from a different culture will encourage readers hopeful of losing some weight themselves to give Japanese food a try. Not only will they like it, but they will also be pleasantly surprised by the results in terms of their body's overall health.

■ ■ ■

## ONE-DAY STARTER MENU FOR DIETING

**Breakfast** (total calories: 531)

Two slices of dry toast (preferably pumpernickel, rye, or French)

One soft-boiled or poached egg sprinkled with granulated kelp

One small green salad with natural cheese added. Salad should consist of 1 oz. dark leafy lettuce, 1 oz. cucumber, $1/2$ oz. celery, 1 oz. shredded cheddar cheese, and $1/2$ tsp. each of rice vinegar, canola oil, and granulated kelp

**Lunch** (total calories: 592)

Noodles cooked with chicken and vegetables
Miso soup with tofu and Chinese black mushrooms

**Dinner** (total calories: 453)

Fish baked with vegetables in aluminum foil
Pumpkin boiled with flavorings
Japanese egg drop soup with chicken and carrot

## NOODLES COOKED WITH CHICKEN AND VEGETABLES

14 oz. thick, dried *udon* (Japanese wheat noodles)

7 oz. chicken, boned and with skin removed (to flavor the chicken in advance, combine 1 tsp. *sake* or rice wine with an equal amount of soy sauce; pour over chicken and soak 10 minutes)

2 oz. carrots

6 fresh Chinese black mushrooms of any other kinds of mushrooms (to precook carrot, chicken, and mushrooms: $^3/_4$ cup *dashi*, 1 tsp. soy sauce, and $^1/_2$ tsp. sugar. To make the *dashi*, boil 1 cup fish bones, fish head, or tail in 3 cups water with 1 Tbsp. coarsely granulated kelp for 25 minutes on low heat, covered; strain, cool, combine with soy sauce and sugar and pour over carrot, chicken, and mushrooms.

4 oz. spinach

2 green onions

4 eggs

*Final broth:* 6 cups of *dashi*, 5 Tbsp. soy sauce, 3 Tbsp. *mirin* (sweet rice wine for cooking), and $^1/_2$ tsp. granulated kelp

$^2/_3$ tsp. *Shichimi togarashi* (powdered cayenne pepper mixed with six other spices; available at any big city Japanese or Oriental food market)

*Note:* This recipe was given to me by the Tokyo equivalent of our Julia Child, Ms. Kiyoko Konishi, who put everything into ounces. To convert into cups, use this simple formula: 8 ounces = 1 cup.

Bring 8 cups of water to a boil, then drop in the noodles a little at a time, making sure you separate them from each other with chopsticks or a fork to prevent them from sticking. When the water boils again, add $^1/_2$ cup cold water to check the bubbling action and to prevent the surface of the noodles from becoming too soft and frayed. When water boils again, repeat the procedure twice more, and cook until the noodles are nearly done, for about 11 minutes. (*Note:* The actual cooking time will depend a lot on the thickness of the noodles, so be sure to follow the instructions given on the package. *Do not overcook.* Slightly heat again just before serving.) Pour into a colander, rinse under cold water, and cover with a damp cloth until ready to use.

Cut the chicken into 1-inch squares. Preflavor with soy sauce and *sake* as given in the instructions under ingredients' list.

Cut the carrots crosswise into thin rounds.

Remove the stems from the mushrooms. Carve crisscross design on the tops.

Bring a pan of water to a boil with a pinch of kelp, and cook the spinach about 3 minutes. Drain. Cool under cold water, gently squeeze out the excess liquid, and cut into inch-long strips.

Cut the green onions crosswise into 1-inch lengths.

Boil the carrots in $3/4$ cup *dashi* with $1/2$ tsp. sugar and 1 tsp. soy sauce for about $2^1/_2$ minutes. Then add the chicken and boil another $2^1/_2$ minutes. Last of all, add the mushrooms and boil $1^1/_2$ minutes.

Mix the ingredients for the final broth and bring to a boil. (Consult the simple instructions given in ingredients list for making the *dashi.*) When ready to serve, put ladle full of broth into ceramic bowls. After this add one quarter of the noodles. Next, divide the carrot, chicken, spinach, green onion, and mushrooms evenly among the bowls. Last of all, pour the remaining one quarter of the broth into each bowl.

Place the bowls on a heavy cookie sheet or flat metal tray in the oven at 375°F. Reheat *only* until they start to form bubbles. At this time, remove them from the oven and break an egg into the center of each bowl. Cover all bowls with another flat cookie sheet. (*Note:* A large turkey baster pan with lid, such as the aluminum disposable kind you can buy in most supermarkets, can be used to place the individual ceramic bowls in.) In a minute the eggs will be half done. Transfer bowls to the table, sprinkle with some *shichimi togarashi,* and eat. Serves 4.

*Note:* All of the aforementioned ingredients may be obtained from a Japanese or Oriental food market in bigger cities.

### Miso Soup with Tofu and Chinese Black Mushrooms

$1/_2$ block *tofu* (tofu is obtained by straining the whey from soy milk curd through a cotton cloth. This is a much finer and more delicate textured tofu than the previous one, which is simply unstrained, coagulated soymilk. Tofu comes in dried or frozen blocks known by a variety of names—*koya-dofu, kori-dofu, shimi-dofu,* or *kogori-dofu.*)

4 fresh Chinese black mushrooms, or other types of fresh mushrooms

4 cups *dashi* (see previous recipe's ingredients list for instructions on making)

2 Tbsp. *miso* (buy sweet white *miso* known as *saikyo* miso. Store in an airtight container in your refrigerator. Since *miso* becomes saltier with time, buy only a small amount and use as quickly as possible)

Remove stems from the Chinese black mushrooms and cut their tops into $1/_2$-inch-wide strips. Then dice the *tofu* into small cubes.

Put the mushrooms into the *dashi* and boil. Continue boiling for another minute, then add the *tofu.* Put the *miso* into the ladle and immerse it in the soup and add the *dashi,* a little at a time, to the *miso,* stirring constantly with chopsticks until thoroughly dissolved. Stir the dissolved *miso* back into the pot gradually, making sure there are no lumps. Right after it boils again, remove from the heat. (*Note: Don't overcook!*)

Put hot soup into bowls and eat. Serves 3–4.

*Note:* All of the aforementioned ingredients may be obtained from a Japanese or Oriental food market in bigger cities. Consult the Yellow Pages of your local telephone directory or inquire of any Oriental restaurant the food market nearest you.

### Fish Baked with Vegetables

This method of cooking without oil, freely combining various ingredients, and adding flavor just before eating is the ideal method for those serious about shedding some unwanted pounds. The taste depends on the selection of fish and vegetables.

4 fillets of fish (cod, flounder, or sea bass)

Fish flavoring: $1/2$ tsp. kelp and 4 tsp. *sake* (rice wine).

2 oz. carrots

2 green peppers

$1/2$ small onion

4 fresh Chinese black mushrooms, or other suitable mushrooms

Vegetable flavoring: $1/2$ tsp. kelp

4 sheets aluminum foil, each 10 inches square (for wrapping up all of these ingredients)

$1/2$ lemon, cut into wedges, or sliced, as condiment

Preheat oven to 320°.

Remove the skin and bones (if any) from the fish and sprinkle each fillet with a pinch of coarsely granulated kelp and 1 tsp. *sake* (dry white wine may be substituted). Let stand for 12 minutes.

Slice the carrots crosswise into thin rounds. If desired, carve the rounds into curious flower shapes.

Remove the seeds from the green peppers, then slice crosswise into thin rings.

Peel the onion and slice it crosswise into thin rounds also.

Remove the stems from the Chinese mushrooms.

Moisten the center of each piece of aluminum foil slightly with *sake* to prevent the fish from sticking. Then put each fish filet and the other ingredients on the foil. Sprinkle with kelp.

Bring the two sides of the foil together above the center of the ingredients and seal by folding down twice in consecutive one-half-inch folds, then securing both right and left edges in the same way.

Bake in the oven for 20 minutes.

Serves 4.

### PUMPKIN BOILED WITH FLAVORINGS

1 lb. pumpkin

$1^1/_2$ cups *dashi* or canned chicken stock

$2^1/_2$ tbsps. sugar

$1^1/_2$ Tbsp. soy sauce

1 Tbsp. *mirin* (sweet rice wine for cooking)

Cut the pumpkin in half, remove the seeds, and wash it. Cut into 2-inch squares. Slice off the skin here and there to give the surface a somewhat mottled appearance and to enable the flavor of the *dashi* to seep in.

Put the pumpkin skin side down into a saucepan, add the *dashi*, sugar, and *mirin*. Cover and boil 10 minutes over medium heat. After 5 minutes, gently turn pieces over one by one.

Next add the soy sauce and continue boiling for 10 minutes, turning over once while boiling. *(Note: Don't overcook!)* Serves 3–4.

### JAPANESE EGG DROP SOUP WITH CHICKEN AND CARROT

3 oz. chicken, bones and skin removed (to flavor the chicken in advance: combine pinch of kelp and 1 tsp. *sake* and pour over poultry. Let set 25 minutes)

1 oz. carrots

2 eggs

*Broth:*

4 cups *dashi* (instructions for making it were given in the ingredients list of the very first recipe), plus $^2/_3$ tsp. kelp and 1 tsp. soy sauce.

Dice the chicken and sprinkle with coarsely granulated kelp (a seaweed) and *sake* (or dry white wine).

Next, cut the carrot crosswise into $^1/_4$-inch rounds. Bring a small amount of water containing $^1/_4$ tsp. kelp to a boil; add the carrots and cook 3 minutes before draining.

Mix the egg well, but lightly, with chopsticks or fork. *(Note: Don't beat!)*

Then bring the *dashi* to boil over high heat. Add the salt, soy sauce, and chicken pieces quickly one by one. Reduce the heat and boil 2 minutes. Add the egg, little by little, stirring always. The soup must be boiling at this stage. When the final egg threads have formed, remove from heat and set aside.

Place the carrots into each soup bowl and pour the hot soup over them. Serves 2–3.

# ADDITIONAL QUICK WEIGHT-LOSS DIETS BASED ON THE ORIENTAL 7-DAY PLAN

■ ■ ■

**I** f you really want to remain slender for the rest of your life and never again worry about putting on weight, you can with the Oriental quick weight-loss rice diet. However, it does entail a strong will, and you have to use many dietary tricks to keep your taste buds happy while going into these various diets.

A predominantly rice diet, either white or brown rice, with plenty of vegetables is the basis of the Oriental system for losing weight. There are variations to the rice diet, however, that you may want to apply from time to time.

Many years ago, when I first became interested in the Oriental system of losing weight and remaining slender, I remember reading an article written by a famous author in a national magazine. He told of how he suffered for years from being overweight, with the usual symptom of high blood pressure and other side effects. He came across the Oriental rice diet, with the addition of vegetables, vitamins, and minerals, and went on this diet, with no meat, and drinking skim milk. He told of how he lost many pounds, how his blood pressure returned to normal, and how he was able to do more work than ever before. Despite years of previous dietary abuses, he lived to be nearly ninety years of age and never again put on the undesired pounds during the rest of his life.

Men like George Bernard Shaw and Mahatma Gandhi were on a similar diet most of their lives and were slender, vital, and youthful in appearance and had tremendous energy throughout their lives.

Heart trouble and high blood pressure are the modern killers in America today. Many doctors have subscribed to the rice diet to help those afflicted with these diseases.

Although rice diets were used by physicians primarily to treat high-blood-pressure cases, it was soon found that these diets had a wonderful side effect. Even though the patients consumed as much as 2,400 calories a day, they did not gain weight.

Before embarking on these stringent diet plans to lose weight, you should always check with your doctor to see that you have no special conditions that make the diet harmful. Then, when on the sustaining, predominantly rice diet, be sure you take one or two vitamin tablets a day, and as most vitamin tablets today contain the required amounts of minerals and other elements, you need not fear that you will become undernourished or sick.

■ ■ ■

## THE FIRST ALL-RICE VARIATION DIET

This Oriental diet is the most stringent of all and should be used by any person who has twenty or more pounds to remove. If you want to lose the weight quickly, you can start this all-rice diet and expect to shed the unwanted pounds more quickly than if you use the rice, fruits, vegetables, and some meat diets given at the beginning of this book.

Prepare your brown rice in advance, and if you cannot buy brown rice in your grocery store, use white rice. Cook it thoroughly, using no salt. (If you cannot stand the thought of saltless food, use the artificial salt that can be found at most markets.) As real salt often holds pounds of water in the body cells, it is a good idea to rid yourself of the salt habit in general, even when you are on the sustaining diet later, when you are permitted to add a variety of other foods to this basic rice diet.

During the day you can eat this rice whenever you feel hungry, three to six times a day. There is a built-in safety feature in this diet—*you can never eat too much rice!* You will not crave excessive amounts, but while on this quick weight-loss diet, you will always feel full, never hungry. This is its great value.

You may drink ten ounces of fruit juice during the day, at any time that you feel thirsty. This can be with the morning meal, or between meals. This can be any kind of fruit juice.

You may have five ounces of any fruits you choose, preferably fresh and in season (to be eaten at or between meals).

You can eat as much as a third of a pound of rice during the day, whenever you feel you are hungry. The rice can be given a variety of tastes by adding pineapple juice to it, a bit of butter, or a small spoonful of honey.

You can drink all the water you want, and all the coffee or tea, with artificial sugar and cream; you can also add two glasses of skim milk, to be taken between meals if you should be hungry.

This stringent rice diet should be taken without any vegetables whatsoever. It cannot harm you if it is indulged in only for a period of three to four weeks. Remember, two-thirds of the people on earth subsist on a predominantly rice diet, and they are slender, have fewer diseases than Americans, and have enough energy to nearly conquer the world in war!

The wonderful thing about this drastic rice diet is that it will melt away at least twelve pounds the first week and possibly as many as fifteen to twenty pounds in the next two weeks. Then you can stop this drastic plan and go on the sustaining diet, which will help you maintain your normal weight.

And remember, if you worry about a lack of protein in this diet, if you eat brown rice instead of processed white rice, you will be obtaining protein and other nourishing elements in the brown rice that will give you many extra benefits.

■ ■ ■

## THE SECOND VARIATION RICE DIET

In this plan you combine the brown or white rice with reducing vegetables, fruit, and fruit juices, but little else.

This diet plan is for those who wish to lose only ten pounds or less, and who may not want to keep up the diet for more than a period of two weeks. It can also be used by those who want to lose from twenty to fifty pounds and who are willing to continue the 7-day plan for several additional weeks.

You can eat any of the following reducing vegetables on this reducing diet, and eat large portions, without fear of putting on pounds. The reason for this, as stated before, is that *these vegetables require more calories to digest than any they give to the body. You cannot overeat them.*

This diet assures you of always feeling comfortably full, and you need not worry about calories, for you will not be adding to your weight on these reducing, low-calorie vegetables.

### The Power-Pack Reducing Vegetables

Following are the vegetables you can eat in any quantities while on these predominantly rice diets without gaining one single ounce of weight. Use these vegetables with the second variation diet, and also with the third diet.

| | | |
|---|---|---|
| string beans | leeks | sauerkraut |
| broccoli | kohlrabi | tomatoes |
| cucumbers | green peppers | turnips |
| celery | lettuce | watercress |
| cabbage | mushrooms | radishes |
| asparagus | spinach | okra |
| garlic | dill pickles | brussels sprouts |
| lettuce | | |

### The Power-Pack Reducing Fruits

You may use these fruits on all three diet plans, as they are reducing fruits and will not upset the reducing plan.

cantaloupe
pumpkin
honeydew melon
watermelon
rhubarb (sweetened with artificial sugar only)

On variation diet number two, you may take the following at every meal:

8 oz. of fruit juice

4 oz. of fruits (but if you take the reducing fruits you can increase this, as these fruits do not add weight, requiring more calories to digest than they give to the body)

All the steamed vegetables you desire in the above list (you may season the vegetables with artificial salt and a little butter)

$1/_3$ lb. of brown rice, with pineapple juice for flavor, or use butter

*Do not* try to eat all the rice at one meal, for you will find doing so difficult, if not impossible. Spread this one third pound of rice over four, or even five meals. You can skip it for breakfast, if you choose, and eat fruits and drink juices with your coffee or tea. Then in mid-morning you can take a portion of vegetables in the reducing list, with a bowl of warmed-up rice. It will keep you from getting hungry all morning.

You may also drink beverages that are low in sugar, such as the dietetic drinks. Eat no fried food on these variation rice diets, and avoid all desserts, outside of the permitted fruits. Be sure to take a therapeutic vitamin while on these rice variation diets.

■ ■ ■

## THE THIRD VARIATION RICE DIET, FOR SLOWER REDUCING RESULTS

This next variation rice diet will also cause you to lose weight steadily, and it gives a little more variety for your taste buds, but is does add more calories, for it includes fish and all varieties of lean meat, except pork. The meats must all be broiled and all fat cut off.

For this variation diet, each day you can add to the second variation rice diet a four-ounce portion of ground round steak, broiled; a piece of veal or beef; a small steak, broiled; or any of the following fish, which are very low in calories:

sea bass
cod steak
flounder
raw oysters
salmon, boiled
fresh tuna
abalone
shrimp, boiled or canned
shad roe

The following meats may be added for this third variation diet, as they are low-calorie foods. Excessive amounts, however, can quickly put the unwanted pounds back on, so use only small portions of about four ounces of these meats.

ground chuck (all fat removed)
filet mignon
heart
kidney
liver
ground round
pot roast
sirloin steak, broiled
sweetbreads
T-bone steak
tenderloin steak
tripe
lamb (lean)
lamb chops, lean
leg of veal or veal cutlets, roasted, with fat removed

One this third variation diet, you can also add the following low-calorie dairy foods. You will still lose weight, but not as rapidly as on the first and second variation rice diets.

cottage cheese
skim milk
buttermilk
yogurt

You may also use eggs in this third variation rice diet—you may eat a poached egg on rice for breakfast, or you may have an egg a day if you decide you do not want to eat the meat and fish on this diet.

You may also add variety to this third rice diet by using any of the following fowl, being sure the skin, where most of the fat is to be found, is removed.

broiled chicken, without stuffing
roast turkey
Cornish hen
pheasant

While on any of these three variation rice diets avoid all of the following high-calorie fattening foods. This applies only to the period of dieting. When you have achieved your desired weight, you may add portions of these foods. They should always be used with great caution, however, for they are high in calories.

cube steak
hamburger
porterhouse steak
rib roast
swiss steak
tongue
boiled or fresh ham
fried lamb chops
roast lamb

■ ■ ■

## THE FOURTH VARIATION RICE DIET

This diet is recommended for those who want to lose very little weight and might even be used as a sustaining diet, when you have lost your desired amount of weight. It is a diet that adds much more variety to your meals and may be taken indefinitely to keep your weight normal.

Keep on eating the brown rice, a little at each meal. This fills you up and makes you want less of the fattening foods, especially the carbohydrates, sugars, and starches.

At each meal eat as much as you want of the fruits and vegetables given in the list of power-pack reducing vegetables. Eat any of the fruits given in the reducing list. Add to your daily diet lean meats, chicken, turkey, fish, cottage cheese, yogurt, and skim milk. Avoid smoked fish or smoked meats while on this diet. Also avoid pork, ham, sausage, herring, salt, ketchup, pickles, relishes, and chili sauce.

While on any of these variation rice diets to lose weight, be sure to avoid all of the following foods. When you have lost the undesired pounds you may use them at your discretion, always remembering that they are the foods that put the weight on you in the first place.

| | |
|---|---|
| candies | gravies |
| cookies | mayonnaise |
| cakes | fatty meats |
| ice cream | meat pies |
| cornstarch | all oils |
| crackers | popcorn |
| high-calorie salad dressings | sundaes |
| fried eggs | sugar |
| fried meats of all kinds | syrup |
| hominy grits | pretzels |
| banana fritters | white breads |
| pancakes and waffles | fatty soups |

The following alcoholic beverages should be avoided while on this reducing plan:

| | | |
|---|---|---|
| beer | cognac | vermouth |
| ale | gin | vodka |
| brandy | rum | whiskey |
| champagne | sherry | dry wine |
| sweet wine | | |

# CHAPTER 9

# THE "VITALIC" SUSTAINING DIET TO KEEP WEIGHT OFF FOR THE REST OF YOUR LIFE

T he big fear that most people have after they have gone through the prolonged agony of losing weight is that it will come right back on again in a matter of a few weeks.

This is apt to be true if you return to your old habits of eating. The important thing to remember is that dieting can be maintained throughout your life without your suffering any harmful effects. Simply cut out the fat-calorie foods in your sustaining diet and replace them with low-calorie foods. In his chapter we shall examine the vitalic sustaining diet that will keep you perfectly nourished without adding extra pounds for the rest of your life.

In any sustaining diet you use try to keep all fat intake to a minimum. It is true that you need some fat each day, but it should be limited to about 60 grams a day. Most diets contain from 250 to 450 grams of fat each day. Any wonder that the body absorbs this unneeded fat and converts it into unwanted pounds?

It is the high fat intake in the average American diet that leads to the deadly effects of cholesterol in the blood.

Hal T., a man whom I once knew, loved to eat fat meats. He would start his day with bacon and eggs; at lunch he ate meat again, with the fat left on it. His wife told me he would even take the fat off her plate at dinner if she did not eat it.

Besides this heavy fat intake, this man was a heavy egg eater, usually having two or three at breakfast. He often varied this with several pancakes with butter and syrup, and as many as three or four pork sausages.

This man was forty-five years of age when he had his first heart attack. When I heard of it, I knew the reason. His cholesterol level had undoubtedly been so increased by his fat consumption that it affected his heart and blood pressure.

Hal weight 220 pounds when he had his heart attack, and his doctor told him he would have to go on a rigid diet to save his life. Fortunately, Hal took this advice seriously. It was at this time that his wife sought me out to find out if he should go on the yoga diet, which I was then giving to thousands of my lecture members and class students at Carnegie Hall.

Hal began this Oriental system of dieting by reducing all fat intake immediately. He used the vegetable reducing soup, the brown rice, some vegetable fat in his salad dressings, and a four-ounce piece of meat twice a day. The brown rice gave him such a feeling of sastisfaction that he soon grew accustomed to going without excess fat. He had been eating as much as 500 grams of fat a day but now on the Oriental diet he was taking less than 60 grams a day. After the first week of fasting and dieting, Hal lost 15 pounds, and then in the succeeding weeks he lost from 15 to 20 pounds a week, until he was down to 180 pounds, which was normal for his age and height. Hal's blood pressure dropped to normal, and he had no recurrence of heart attacks in the next two years I observed him.

■ ■ ■

## THE VITALIC FOODS THAT DO NOT PUT ON WEIGHT

Following are the foods you can eat the rest of your life that will keep you from putting on those extra pounds in the future. Most of these foods are in the regular Oriental quick-loss diet, but now we shall add foods that give more low-fat calories as well as good nutrition.

### The Value of Soups as Fillers

You can still take one or two bowls of soup a day while on the sustaining diet. However, now that the unwanted pounds are gone, you can switch from the power-pack reducing vegetables that add no calories, taking instead regular soups made with vegetables and lean meats. Be sure to skim off all fats that gather on such soups.

You can use vegetable broths and cream soups, but let the cream be skim milk.

Add to the sustaining diet the nourishing legume family to prepare your soups. Lentils are an excellent source of nourishment without adding fats. Cook the lentils with one large onion chopped up, artificial salt, and a small amount of polyunsaturated corn oil. (Remember, the body requires at least two tablespoons of fat or oil a day, so do not eliminate fat entirely from your cooking while on this sustaining diet.)

Make soups also from dried peas and navy beans. In the pea soup, as well as the lentil soup, you can add cut-up pieces of lean frankfurters. Be sure they are beef, not pork. This soup can be eaten for luncheon, with a small green salad, tea or coffee, and a gelatin dessert, made with artificial sugar. You will feel full, and yet your body will not absorb many calories from this luncheon.

■ ■ ■

## LARGE VARIETY OF MEATS POSSIBLE WITH SUSTAINING DIET

Unfortunately, all meats, even when lean, have veins of fat in them. As meats are desirable forms of protein for any sustaining diet, it is important that you choose those that are lean and prepare them in such a way that the fat will be cooked out.

If you use ground round or chuck, ask the butcher to trim all excess fat away.

Avoid frying all meats in oil from now on, for this is one of the ways by which you absorb many fat calories that quickly bring back the unwanted pounds. You can instead fry meat without using fat in the pan. Sprinkle a little salt in the heated pan, put the meat in, and turn it several times until cooked well.

A couple of products are now on the market that are recommended for low-fat cooking of meat or eggs. These are sprayed onto the frying pan, and then the meat or eggs are cooked in it. The food will not stick to the pan.

Avoid the high-fat and -cholesterol meats such as pork chops, roast loin of pork, bacon, and ham. The same thing applies to sausage, salami, liverwurst, brains, kidneys, and sweetbreads. You can eat small quantities of these foods once a week to add variety to the diet, but generally they should be avoided if you want to keep away from the high-calorie foods.

Liver is usually excellent and can be broiled or fried in the above manner, without use of fat.

To add to the appeal of your meat dishes while on the permanent sustaining diet, you can garnish them with various types of fruits. If you use canned fruits be sure to wash out the excess sugars that are contained in the syrup. These add hundreds of unwanted calories and should be avoided. You can use sliced pineapple, purple plums, peach halves, prunes, or broiled bananas.

A good way to add variety to meat dishes is through the use of various sauces, such as chili sauce, ketchup, relishes, jellies, applesauce, mint jelly, cranberry sauce, and chutney.

Also, to keep meats from tasting uniformly the same try adding herbs and spices to your cooking, such as garlic, basil, oregano, thyme, and bay leaves. Greek and Italian dishes frequently use these spices, especially oregano, to enliven their cooked meats, and spices add nothing in the way of calories.

■ ■ ■

## USE POULTRY OF ALL KINDS TO ADD TASTY PROTEINS

Your sustaining diet will vary greatly if you do not restrict yourself to the well-known meats. Use chicken, turkey, and squab or Guinea hen occasionally to give variety to your meat intake. If most of the fat is cooked out of the turkey or chicken in baking, rather than frying, fewer calories will be added. Duck is filled with too much fat, as is goose, but for variety small portions of these can be eaten once in a while without upsetting the diet.

You can also use chicken and turkey for sandwiches and salads, with a low-calorie mayonnaise. Be sure that you use the protein breads or the whole-wheat breads, and avoid white breads, which have had all the nourishment processed out of them. An excellent lunch on this sustaining diet can be a chicken or turkey sandwich, with a small salad, a glass of milk, or coffee or tea; or a chicken or turkey salad with a low-calorie mayonnaise.

### *Fish Dishes Best Source of Protein on the Sustaining Diet*

Many nutritionists now claim that many types of fish are better protein sources, with less fat, than some of the meat proteins. However, if fish is fried, fat calories are unnecessarily added. It is best to broil fresh fish, without the use of oil.

Flounder, perch, scallops, haddock, and sturgeon are all excellent forms of protein with very little fat. You can eat small portions of fish like brook trout, porgy, cod, and croakers, but they are a little higher in fat calories than the former.

Lobster, crabs, and shrimp are exceedingly low in fat calories and cholesterol content. Clams are also excellent if eaten raw or in a stew. Fried, they become saturated in fat calories. Oysters are also excellent eaten raw or in stews.

Tuna fish, fresh or canned, is generally low in fat calories, although some brands of tuna, when packed in oil, do not fit into this category. Choose the brands that are not packed in oil. Sardines are high in fat calories and should be eaten on a day when your fat intake from other meals has been below average.

■ ■ ■

## THE VALUE OF MILK PRODUCTS IN YOUR DIET

It used to be thought that adults didn't require milk after their teeth and bones had matured. Now the latest scientific research shows that milk is really good for everybody, no matter what age. The only thing that should be avoided by most people is the high cholesterol of the fat in milk. But today, with skim milk, or low-fat milk, fortified, we can safely take at least one pint of milk a day. Milk contains many valuable proteins, and when it is used with additional amounts of vitamins A and D that fortify the milk, it becomes a highly nutritious food. You can also take buttermilk occasionally to add variety.

A very good, quick way to build energy when you feel a sense of fatigue due to lowered blood sugar is to fortify a glass of skim milk with two tablespoons of dried milk. This enriches the skim milk and makes it more palatable.

You can also use yogurt that is made from nonfat milk. This adds to the body's nutrition without giving you too many fat calories. However, it must be remembered that yogurt is assimilated easily without much work for the stomach, and all such foods add more calories than do those that the stomach has to work hard to digest. So do not feel you can eat all the yogurt you want, without adding some fattening calories.

■ ■ ■

## WHAT ABOUT CHEESE PRODUCTS?

Few cheeses fit in any sustaining diet if they are eaten in large quantities, for most cheeses are high in butterfat content. This includes cheese dips and cheese spreads of all kinds. If you are at a party, however, and these are served, you can safely eat a few if you have restricted your high-calorie foods for that day in other departments.

Cottage cheese or pot cheese can be used in your sustaining diet if it is made from nonfat milk. Most cottage cheese must contain a certain amount of butterfat to meet federal regulations. Check your brand of cottage cheese to be sure that it does not contain excessive amounts of butterfat. Many people make this error in dieting—they eat all the cottage cheese they want, never knowing that unless it is the low-butterfat type it is *not* a good food for losing weight.

■ ■ ■

## THE VALUE OF VEGETABLES IN THE MAINTENANCE DIET

The list of vegetables given for the vegetable soup and the power-pack reducing vegetables may all be eaten in any sustaining diet. However, when you want to maintain a well-balanced diet you can also add other vegetables, such as peas, carrots, corn and potatoes.

The ideal way to use vegetables of course, is by eating them raw in nourishing salads. If vegetables are cooked in the usual manner by boiling, many of their nutritive elements are destroyed and they are useless to the body. The best way to prepare most vegetables is by steaming them until tender. Cook them with artificial salt, and no oil or fat. Instead of using butter or other fats try using a bouillon cube or some herbs to add to the taste. Avoid creamed sauces, or heavy butter. If you want a little margarine to add to the flavor, heat it and pour it over the steamed vegetables just before serving.

Later we shall learn how you can be a vegetarian, if you want to adopt a meatless diet and still not suffer from protein starvation.

■ ■ ■

## FRUITS—NATURE'S SWEET DESSERTS

Many people who go through the rigors of a diet to lose from ten to fifty pounds complain because most desserts are denied to them while dieting. As a heavy carbohydrate eater misses her sugars, starches, and fats more than anything else in her restrictive reducing diet, it is important that your sustaining diet supply you with some sweets.

Fruits, and desserts made from fruits, are the best way for you to obtain your sugars. As there is no fat in fruits, you never need to worry about cholesterol in a heavy fruit diet. However, if you overeat even of fruits, you will soon find yourself putting the unwanted pounds back on again, for fruits are full of natural sugars, when taken in excess, and sugars always put on weight.

Dates and figs are high in sugars, but make good, tasty substitutes for candy, cakes, and pies. Prunes are also highly nutritive and fill you up quickly. Eat all the apples, cantaloupes, watermelon, cherries, and strawberries you want when they are in season, for these are on the list of fruits that take more calories to digest than they give to your body. Avoid syrups and too much honey, as these are rich in carbohydrates and are converted into fat without much effort by the body.

Eat oranges and pineapples and most other fruits whole, rather than the juices from them, for it takes the stomach longer to digest them whole and uses up most of the calories in the digestive process. Most fruits can be used diet without restriction while on your sustaining diet, and they make excellent sources of quick sugar for between-meal snacks.

Tasty fruit salads can be eaten for lunch or dinner. However, it is best to avoid eating citrus fruits when you eat starch foods, such as bread, corn, or peas. As these two have chemical digestions, starches and acids should not be eaten at the same meal.

Another good rule to observe is to avoid eating the high-protein meats at the same time as you eat starches, in breads or vegetables such as corn and peas, or potatoes. Chemical mixtures are not conducive to good digestion when these opposing chemical combinations are eaten in the same meal. This is why many people who are big meat, potato, and bread eaters, topping it off with ice cream, cake, or pie, often suffer from terrific indigestion and gas attacks later. These foods require different chemicals to digest. Starches digest predominantly in the mouth, whereas proteins digest in the stomach.

■ ■ ■

## WOMAN WITH CHRONIC INDIGESTION CURED

Mabel P. was not only overweight when she first came to see me, but she complained of chronic indigestion. She said doctors had found nothing wrong with her, and she accepted this as a cross she had to bear.

In our first consultation I asked her to give me the typical day's food intake she was following. She told me in detail what her diet had been, and it was apparent why she suffered from gas, heartburn, and chronic indigestion. She was mixing her starches and proteins and acids indiscriminately at all her meals! For instance, at breakfast she took a glass of orange juice, which was fine, but on top of the orange juice she ate a starchy cereal or two eggs with white toast (more starch), and then coffee with cream and sugar. The starches and sugars simply did not mix with the proteins, such as eggs and milk, or with the acids, represented by the orange juice or other citrus fruits.

At lunch she ate more meat; potatoes, and white bread (more starch); and sometimes a fruit dessert, or jello with fruit, or sometimes a fruit yogurt. This mixture of fruit acids with starches and proteins made an indigestible combination, as the starches digest predominantly in the mouth, while the meats and fruits digest in the stomach and intestines.

The moment Mabel began to eat her proteins and fruits together, and her starches alone, she lost all signs of indigestion! In the morning she drank her orange juice half an hour before her regular meal, and she suffered no further discomfort.

■ ■ ■

## SALADS—THE BUFFER FOODS TO KEEP YOU FROM OVEREATING

It is difficult to overeat of salads, for they furnish so much bulk that a person can hardly overeat these valuable foods. All kinds of fruits and vegetables may be used in making up salads that will be helpful on your sustaining diet in giving you that satisfied, full feeling, and yet furnishing you with valuable minerals and other elements you require.

Salad dressings are the big danger in the reducing diet as well as in the maintenance diet that follows. It is always wise to avoid the high-fat content of the salad dressings on the market and to favor those that are low in fat. Many of these salad dressings are on the market, and they should be used from now on.

In making up your salads be sure to use raw vegetables as much as possible. You can add fresh fruits to appetizing salads, and to fill out your list of salads you might try combining cottage cheese and gelatin. When you cannot get fresh fruits do not be afraid to use canned fruits, being sure you wash off the excess sugar that comes in the thick syrup.

Following are some tasty recipes that utilize salads that can be served for a complete lunch, or added to the dinner menu with meats and other vegetables.

### Grapefruit and Asparagus Salad

Use canned asparagus when you cannot get it fresh

2 grapefruits

Salad greens

1 green pepper

Cut grapefruit into segments, removing all seeds. Put the asparagus stalks on individual plates that have first been prepared with salad greens. Put about 5 or 6 stalks of asparagus on each plate, with the slices of grapefruit arranged to alternate with the asparagus. Cut the green pepper into slender strips and place a strip alongside each stalk of asparagus or across it. Add special reducing dressing and serve.

### Coleslaw Salads

Coleslaw prepared in various ways can add a tasty variety to salad menus, especially when prepared with oranges, apples, cucumbers, or pineapple.

To prepare the basic coleslaw, use a slaw cutter or very sharp knife to shred the cabbage. Avoid the tough outer leaves, and using the inner tender leaves only. Wash the cabbage thoroughly, and after it has been shredded, add minced onion and parsley sprigs, and also $3/4$ cup of special low-fat dressing.

To add variety to the above coleslaw recipe add the following ingredients:

*Apple Coleslaw:* Chop up 2 large apples, without the skin, and cut up 2 pimentos. Add this to the above coleslaw.

*Orange Coleslaw:* Cut two oranges into segments and then divide them into smaller pieces, and add to the basic coleslaw recipe above.

*Pineapple Coleslaw:* Remove the onion from the above basic coleslaw and add 1 cup of shredded canned pineapple, or fresh pineapple if available.

*Cucumber Coleslaw:* Use 1 large cucumber. Chop it up and add it to the basic coleslaw.

### APPLE, RAISIN, AND WALNUT SALAD

Another good combination for a tasty salad uses apples, raisins, and walnuts.

To prepare this salad use a large salad bowl into which you rub a cut clove of garlic, or you may use a half spoonful of garlic salt. Put a teaspoon of mustard in the bowl. Add a tablespoon of salad oil (polyunsaturated oil is preferred to olive oil, although for better taste you may use olive oil). Stir the oil and mustard together, then add 2 tablespoons of lemon juice, and blend all together.

Add freshly cut-up lettuce leaves, uncooked garden peas, small cut-up carrots, peeled cut-up tomatoes, and watercress. Use quartered hard-boiled eggs for garnishing the dish.

To the above basic salad add shredded white cabbage, chopped apples, seedless raisins and chopped walnuts. Mix with your favorite low-calorie salad dressing and serve.

You may use the above basic salad bowl to prepare a variety of other tasty and nutritious salads.

### BEAN SPROUT SALAD

A delicious bean sprout salad can be made as follows:

Use a cupful of bean sprouts, either fresh or canned. Add to this $1/4$ cucumber that you dice, $1/2$ cup of chutney sauce, and 1 cup of pineapple cubes. Garnish this with sliced tomatoes and halved hard-boiled eggs. You can further decorate the salad bowl with strips of red pimentos or red and green peppers. Add all these ingredients to the basic lettuce salad given previously.

### DATE, GINGER, AND BANANA SALAD

Serve on a bed of lettuce the following ingredients: quartered bananas, cut up lengthwise; dates from which the pit has been removed; and artificial whipped-cream dressings, sprinkled lightly with shredded ginger.

### CREAM CHEESE AND PINEAPPLE SALAD

This is a tasty variation on regular salads and is a complete lunch if served with date nut bread or whole-wheat bread.

Put several pineapple slices on a bed of lettuce, and heap cream cheese on the lettuce leaves. Use finely ground nuts over it. No salad dressing is required for this.

### PEAR, PEPPER, AND CHICORY SALAD

Serve this in the basic salad bowl given above. Blend chicory pieces and quarters of fresh, ripe pear (or canned), with thin strips of green pepper, and serve on bed of lettuce, with a low-calorie dressing.

### TOMATO SALADS

Stuffed tomato salads are always eye-appealing as well as healthful and nutritious for any sustaining diet.

You can stuff tomatoes with a variety of foods, such as small shrimp, crab, chopped-up lobster tails, creamed mushrooms, hard-boiled eggs, cream cheese, chopped nuts, and nutmeat mixtures.

Cut the tops off the ripe tomatoes and take out the center pulp, blending it with the various ingredients given above.

■ ■ ■

## THE USE OF CEREALS IN THE SUSTAINING DIET

Part of the value of any sustaining diet, after the undesired weight has been lost, is to add to the future eating habits those foods that give nourishment, variety, and necessary nutrients, without danger of putting back unwanted pounds that have been lost.

Most cereals are carbohydrates, it is true, but they are also virtually fat-free. As some carbohydrates are essential to any balanced, sustaining diet, you can use whole-wheat cereals, bran, corn flakes, oat products such as oatmeal, grits, and hominy, with additions of stewed or canned fruits or fresh fruits like bananas and berries in season. Also prunes, peaches, pears, apricots, figs, dates, and raisins may be added for tasty variety to the cereals.

Whole-wheat grains are also important because they contain the vitamin-B complex and also proteins. Many people like to add wheat germ to their breakfast cereals. Cooked cereals may be cooked with skim milk rather than whole milk.

A good solid breakfast is important to any sustaining diet and may include a cereal, cold or hot, with skim milk; an egg, poached, or cooked without fat; with bacon, or ham. Fruit, such as orange or grapefruit, berries, or other fruits in season make for a complete breakfast, with the addition of coffee or tea, using artificial sugar and real cream.

■ ■ ■

## A WOMAN WHO SKIPPED BREAKFASTS TO REDUCE SUFFERED FATIGUE

Ruth I. was twenty-four years of age, and weighed 155 pounds when she began to be serious about losing weight. She had tried drastic reducing methods and sometimes lost the desired weight, but it kept coming back. She tried skipping breakfasts entirely, usually drinking two cups of black coffee, and then having her lunch at the office restaurant, where she was so famished she usually overate of sandwiches and sweets.

When she began the Oriental reducing diet, she suffered from chronic headaches, irritability, and nervousness. Her doctor found nothing organically wrong with her, but did tell her she must lost some weight, as her normal weight for her height and age should have been 130 pounds.

The first thing I urged Ruth to do in approaching her new Oriental reducing plan was to eat a big breakfast. This amazed her, as she did not realize that lowered blood sugar in the early-morning hours often causes symptoms such as she had, and leads to a desire to overeat at lunch.

She ate two eggs, poached, and two slices of thoroughly cooked bacon, a slice of whole-wheat toast with butter, and real cream in her coffee. She needed some fats, and the cream and butter gave her some of the required daily intake she needed to improve her metabolism.

The breakfast she ate kept her from being famished at lunch, and she satisfied her protein needs with slices of ham or beef, cheddar cheese, and a fruit for dessert.

For her dinners Ruth had a wide variety of choices according to our Oriental food plan. With rice as the staple, she satisfied her craving for carbohydrates and sugars and soon was tipping the scales at 140 pounds. It took her only three weeks to shed the full 25 pounds, and this she did without ever feeling hungry or suffering from the former symptoms of fatigue, irritability, and nervousness.

# Built-in Safety Features in the 7-Day Oriental Quick Weight-Loss Diet

■ ■ ■

The objections that most physicians and nutritionists have to the usual quick weight-loss diets is that these diets are unbalanced, failing to supply the body with the vitamins, minerals, and other elements that are required to keep it at its peak of efficiency.

To reassure yourself on that score, you can know that the built-in safety features of this diet will prevent you from suffering anything negative to your health.

Consider a few facts that have been observed by scientists regarding stringent dietary deficiencies, under forced conditions. Many people who have gone on hunger strikes for many days were found to suffer from great weight loss but few other physical symptoms. During most of our major wars, when prisoners were put on diets that were close to starvation diets, it was found that they suffered less from heart disease, high blood pressure, and other diseases that usually are thought to be associated with dietary deficiencies. In fact, these prisoners not only suffered from insufficient nourishment, but they were usually in the most unsanitary condition, they were often tortured and relentlessly questioned, giving added mental stress, and yet they survived these long terms of imprisonment without succumbing to fatal illnesses.

During World War II in Europe, most of the people lacked meats, fats, proteins, vitamins, and other foods considered essential to a balanced diet. These thousands upon thousands of people did not collapse from these limitations in their diets. In fact, they seemed to actually become healthier on their reduced diets! They suffered less from diseases of the heart, hypertension, gallbladder disorders, and many other diseases that had formerly killed them by the thousands.

During the Nazi invasions of Holland and Norway, when the populations were practically on starvation diets, hospital admissions dropped 40 percent over periods when the populations were considered well fed and well nourished.

The moment the war ended and people could obtain all the usual foods things changed again. By 1949 the rate of heart disease, high blood pressure, and other diseases returned to the same levels as before the war. This proved that people suffer more illnesses from being overfed than from diets that contain some restrictions and limitations over a period of a few weeks.

However, for those who have such fears about reducing diets of any kind, I shall give you some built-in safety features that you may observe during the times you are on the Oriental 7-day reducing plan. You will then be assured of the fact that you are obtaining all the essential vitamins, minerals, and other elements that scientists and nutrition experts agree should be in every balanced diet to maintain the body at its peak of health and energy, even during periods of strenuous reducing.

Despite the fact that Americans are considered the best-fed people in the world, most nutrition experts agree that our diets are deficient in most of the important elements of nutrition. If this can occur when we are not dieting to lose weight, how much more can it be said for most reducing diets, which deprive a person of so many foods that are considered essential to a balanced diet?

■ ■ ■

## SUPPLEMENTS TO THE ORIENTAL 7-DAY DIET

To avoid these deficiencies and dangers while on your reducing diet, and later, while on the sustaining normal diet, you can begin immediately to add certain vitamins, minerals, and other essential elements that are considered vital to good nutrition.

Follow this regimen to the letter if you want to gain immeasurable benefits from these dietary supplements while you are on your reducing diet and long after, for the rest of your natural life. These steps will assure you of being fortified with essential protections so you will never again suffer from nutritional deficiencies.

**1.** Be sure to include in your reducing diet, and in the sustaining diet after you have lost your desired amount of weight, the important B-complex vitamins each day. Two tablets generally contain the essential B vitamins, but you should check the label or consult your physician to see that you are taking the required amounts of the right vitamins for your personal needs.

The metabolization of carbohydrates requires thiamine or $B_1$. This also helps you break down sugars in the diet to give you energy. Lack of this vitamin produces fatigue, nausea, psychic and emotional disturbances, poor appetite, and sometimes sensations of numbness and very often moodiness and depression. Also, lack of this vitamin sometimes produces leg pains.

The B-complex vitamins also include riboflavin, or $B_2$; niacin; pyridoxine, or $B_6$; and $B_{12}$.

If these vital elements are lacking in your diet you will have symptoms of every known type of disorder. This vital information is given fully in Chapter 6 of this book, and you should study it carefully again, to be sure you are not missing out on all of these vital vitamins.

**2.** Each day use a very important food supplement that has lately been discovered, and is considered to be in the nature of a miracle worker—this is lecithin, an extract made from soybeans.

Lecithin can be added to breakfast cereals, using from two to four tablespoonsful, which will give you enough of this vital element for the entire day.

Lecithin is a powder made by grinding up soybeans. The soybean was used in the Orient for centuries, and only recently have scientists discovered this miraculous substance it contains.

Lecithin plays an important role in the life function of all living cells, in both animals and humans. It is found in all living cells and plays a big part in the body's correct functioning and in its chemistry.

Scientists found that lecithin was helpful in reducing the cholesterol from the blood vessels in the treatment of heart disease. Injections of lecithin in animals were shown to remove the cholesterol plaque that had been deposited in the arteries.

Other experiments with lecithin in the human diet showed other remarkable results: it was found to help in the metabolizing of fats; it also increases the gamma globulin of the blood, which helps the body resist various infections. Lecithin has also been found useful in the prevention and treatment of many diseases including kidney disorders, metabolic disturbances of the skin such as psoriasis, rheumatic carditis, and diseases of the liver, as well as anemia.

Patients who have been put on this oil-free program of lecithin reported that they felt better in general, had more energy and vitality for their daily work, and were sick less often than formerly.

A case that I personally had contact with, proving the remarkable powers that lecithin has when added to the human diet, was that of a woman who was forty-five years of age, and chronically tired. Brenda W. thought it was a symptom of her change of life, and her physician could find nothing organically wrong. She was about twenty pounds overweight when I first met her, and she told me that her sex life with her husband had deteriorated; she felt no response to his lovemaking and thought there was something wrong with her.

After she had been on the Oriental diet for about two weeks, she lost her undesired weight, but still felt no desire for lovemaking with her husband.

It was then that I remembered the remarkable effects that the addition of lecithin to the food plan had had on other people and I told her about the added sexual vigor as well as untiring energy that these people had known after two or three weeks of taking lecithin and other supplements. She consulted her doctor, who told her to try it, as she was in good physical condition now and it might help her.

When Brenda reported to me three weeks later, I was astounded at the change in her. She walked with a youthful bounce; her eyes were clear and flashed vitality and energy. She told me that after taking about four tablespoons of lecithin powder a day, which she added to her breakfast cereals, she had felt like a youngster again. Her sexual enjoyment came back, and she and her husband began a new relationship that promises happiness for the future.

**3.** Vitamin A and vitamin C have also been found to be highly beneficial in any diet, used daily. The recommended dosages that have been approved are 25,000 units of vitamin A and a minimum of 150 mg. of vitamin C. Many doctors recommended higher dosages; consult your physician to determine your personal requirements.

**4.** A few years ago a famous writer on nutrition recommended a standard formula of blackstrap molasses, wheat germ, skim milk fortified with powdered milk, and yeast as a good daily way to obtain many essential vitamins and minerals. Scientists have often scoffed at this formula, but it has not been disproved. It is still considered by many to be an excellent way in which to obtain essential vitamins and minerals.

**5.** To furnish the body with essential fatty acids, which are required in any balanced daily program of nutrition, it is recommended by many doctors that a person take at least two tablespoonsful of corn oil, safflower oil, or soybean oil daily. Some people make up salad dressings using these oils, and many people take them with tomato juice to make them more palatable.

For centuries people in the Far East have known about the value of soybeans in their diet. This is one of the most valuable sources of unsaturated fatty acids and is thought to be one of the reasons why so many Orientals who follow this type of diet have little heart disease and seldom suffer from arteriosclerosis.

Soybean oil can generally be obtained in food markets and at health food stores. Each tablespoonful of soybean oil contains about 135 calories, and it can easily be used in place of olive oil or the other vegetable oils for salads and for various forms of cooking.

**6.** Obtaining your vitamins and minerals from natural foods is better than taking these in capsule and pill form, of course. One very good way by which you can obtain many of the essential vitamins and minerals is to grow a trayful of wheat sprouts. You can use a tin tray and put sand in it, placing the wheat in the sand, and covering with a damp cloth, giving a little moisture to the seed. In a few days, if you keep the cloth damp, little green shoots will start to come up. When these are one or two inches high, pull them up and wash them. Add them to your salads.

**7.** Many people are deficient in calcium, with resultant fatigue and other negative effects on the body. To avoid making this mistake, even while dieting you should take at least two glasses of skim milk a day, and add to the milk about two tablespoons of powdered milk. This helps give the body necessary proteins and also keeps the calcium level high. Sometimes during dieting, you may feel hungry at two or three in the morning, and this may be due to the fact that your blood sugar has reached low levels. It is then that you need something to eat that will raise the blood sugar level but not add extra fat.

You can put three tablespoonsful of powdered milk into a glass of skim milk and drink this. It will begin to give you the extra energy you will require the next morning when you awaken with that down-in-the-mouth feeling. This is a good practice to follow even when you are on your regular diet, for it keeps you from growing so hungry that you eat more than you should at regular meals.

Martha N. was a lecture member who tried the Oriental reducing diet with great benefits, shedding about thirty-five pounds in a period of a little over three weeks. She reported regularly that she felt fine, except that she seemed not to have the energy she had once known when she was younger. She was only thirty-nine years of age, and with the lost weight she should have felt much better.

I remembered research I had done some years ago on calcium deficiency, which scientists had discovered led to fatigue and other negative symptoms. I told Martha to try adding skim milk (with two tablespoons of powdered milk) to her regular diet. She did this between meals, especially in the morning when she had a very light breakfast. Soon she said she had energy enough to do her regular housework and that the energy lasted until midafternoon, when she took another glass of skim milk with two more tablespoons of powdered milk. In about three weeks' time Martha seemed to be back to normal. She kept up the skim milk and powdered milk as a part of her daily supplement and reported that she had no further trouble with abnormal fatigue.

**8.** If you carry your lunch to work and are on a diet, you can still keep yourself down to the calories you should absorb by adding some of the following nourishing foods to your lunch without fearing that you are adding weight.

You can carry a four-ounce serving of any lean meat, and a small container of salad, with a nonfattening dressing.

Celery stalks, radishes, and olives add taste to such a lunch and are easy to carry. You can add hard-boiled eggs and tomatoes to your lunch, without fearing that your are overindulging in fatty foods. Corned beef slices with lettuce leaves between them also add tasty variety to a luncheon you must eat at work. A fresh apple or orange, or even a fruit compote, can be carried along for dessert. Then at dinner you can carry out the balance of your normal Oriental diet with the vegetables or vegetable soup, and the brown rice.

**9.** You should avoid all alcoholic beverages while on the Oriental diet, for these add many extra calories to your food intake. However, if you have to have a cocktail before dinner or at a social gathering and you feel you must take a drink, you can add one or two cocktails to your daily intake of calories and cut down on the rice for that day or eat fewer calories in your other foods.

**10.** Through the years, I've recommended a number of specific health food products made by a Japanese company for losing weight efficiently and keeping it off for good. These products are distributed in the United States by Wakunaga of America Co., Ltd., of Mission Viejo, California. They form an ideal supplement program to stay healthy and slender by. They are available at most local health food stores. Here is the standard supplement program that many people go on who wish to use these fine products while dieting.

KYO-GREEN Powdered Drink Mix. 1 Tbsp. in 8 oz. of water or juice every morning at breakfast and again in the evening with dinner.

KYOLIC Aged Garlic Extract Super Formula 106 (with vitamin E, cayenne, and hawthorn berry). Take 2 capsules in the morning with breakfast.

KYOLIC Aged Garlic Extract Dietary Supplement Formula 105 (with vitamins A, C, E, and selenium). Take 2 capsules with meals three times daily.

PREMIUM KYOLIC-EPA (marine lipid concentrates and aged garlic extract). Take 2 capsules in the morning with food.

GINGO BILOBA PLUS (with Kyolic Aged Garlic Extract). Take 2 capsules in the evening just before retiring.

KYO-DOPHILUS (for the gastrointestinal tract). Take 1 capsule per meal (twice that amount when traveling in foreign countries). (See Appendix II for more information on obtaining these products.)

■ ■ ■

## A WOMAN WHO DID NOT EXERCISE WEIGHED 210 POUNDS

One hour of the right kind of exercise can often help you get away with a higher caloric intake. If you have gone on a binge and eaten a piece of pie or cake, which is forbidden on your regular diet, you can burn up these extra calories by vigorous exercise for an hour. You can swim, play tennis, walk vigorously, or ride a bicycle for an hour and burn up several hundred calories.

Of course exercise should be indulged in while you are losing weight as well as throughout your lifetime. If you do simple sitting-up exercises a few moments a day you use up only 200 calories an hour—so you cannot eat more just because of this. Exercise has to be vigorous and indulged in daily for an hour or two if you wish to burn up excess calories. Each day walk, swim, play volleyball or tennis, or get some other form of vigorous exercise (being sure to check with your doctor that you have no special condition that forbids such rigorous physical activity) that will assure you of using up several hundred calories per day. You will lose weight much faster in this way than if you do no physical exercise at all.

A woman who came to my lecture work was 210 pounds when she sought me out for an interview. She did not actually come because of her weight—she dismissed that by saying her mother was fat, and it was a hereditary condition, due, no doubt, to her glands. This is an excuse that many fat people rely on. What she did come about was the fact that her husband no longer found her attractive, since she had put on all that excess weight, for she had once been only 140 pounds, and with her big frame and height she could carry that quite well. She wanted to know how to bring her husband back to her, as they had been in earlier years.

In studying her personal habits I found that she sat around all day watching TV and eating in-between-meal snacks, which usually included a box of chocolates a week, and other sugar desserts.

In counseling her, I told her first to see her doctor to learn if she could take a stringent diet, and then I remembered in my travels throughout India I had seen one town where the women were extremely fat, from eating large quantities of sweets, which they made. These women weighed from 190 to 250 pounds, and did no exercise; they just sat around eating sweets.

Then I recalled other tribes in India who were physically very active, the men hunting for their meat, the women tending the crops in the fields, and these people were slender, wiry, and energetic, with not one fat person in the village.

I had to work very hard to get this woman to give up her sweets, but to win her husband's love back she agreed to do so. Then she was put on the most stringent diet using our Oriental method of vegetables and brown rice, with the stipulation that she was not to sit around all day, but rather indulge in some form of exercise. She joined a women's reducing gym, where she was given exercises that fit her needs, and with this form of physical activity and the Oriental diet combined, she lost 15 pounds the first week. Within three months, she had shed the unwanted pounds and was back to 140 pounds. She reported that she felt better than ever before and her husband's romantic interests had been revived.

More recent information given on the ABC program "Good Morning, America" on Thursday, January 18, 1996, showed that if this woman had walked 3 miles per hour she would have burned up 250 calories. Had she walked 5 miles an hour, vigorously swinging her arms and taking long strides (so as to increase her body's metabolic rate), she would have lost 500 calories. Walking is good for you, whether it is done leisurely in a stroll for enjoyment or more vigorously in "power walking" for physical stimulation. It will not only help you to shed unwanted pounds but make you feel good and look great besides!

# HOW TO ADD ZEST TO YOUR ORIENTAL DIET

N■■■

ow you are ready to undertake a study
of the foods you can add to your Oriental diet,
foods that will give zest to your meals without
adding fat calories and that will give you perfect nourishment while you are on the diet
and afterward.

These foods may be eaten after you have
taken off the desired number of pounds and
your weight is normal. They will give you tremendous energy, keep you young longer, and
always keep your weight at normal without
effort on your part.

The following foods will diversify your
Oriental diet, and they will be burned up
quickly by the body, not stored as fat. These
vital foods are not the carbohydrate foods that

put on your weight in the first place, but they are in the protein and fat classification of foods, which give energy but do no put on the excess fat.

The foods in the carbohydrate class, that is, starches and sugars, give joy to the taste buds, for they add pleasure to eating, but they are also the calories that put excess fat on quickly.

The carbohydrate foods are generally high in fat content and are quickly stored by the body as excess fat. These are the well-known desserts, pie, cake, waffles, pancakes, cream sauces, ice cream, cookies, and breads.

If you begin now to eliminate most of these excess carbohydrates from your slenderizing diet and never touch them the rest of your life, it will help you not only in maintaining your perfect weight, but in being healthier, having more energy, and living longer.

I know you will instantly ask: But aren't carbohydrates necessary in the daily diet? To that we can answer: Yes, they are necessary, but only in minute quantities, not in the large amounts most Americans take them in their daily food intake. If you eliminate the above devitalizing carbohydrates and take the Oriental vital list of foods, you will be getting all the carbohydrates you require in your sustaining diet without adding the heavy fat calories represented by starches and sugars.

Breads, potatoes, and sweet desserts are the mainstay of the average American diet. You can safely rid your diet of these forever and suffer only one consequence, being healthier and never again growing fat! Yes, the carbohydrate foods are appealing to the taste buds, but they are harmful to the body, and they put fat on the body that kills.

The Oriental foods, by their wide variety and because they are natural and not devitalized, furnish the body with all the proteins and other elements required to maintain perfect health and keep the body slender and functioning healthfully.

■ ■ ■

## BROWN RICE AND ITS VALUE OVER WHITE RICE

One of the staples in our Oriental diet for reducing without hunger is brown rice. A person may argue that this is a pure carbohydrate food, but he would be wrong. Brown rice contains many other vital food elements besides carbohydrates. It is rich in proteins, and in vitamins and minerals. Only when the natural brown rice has been processed and the coating removed are all the essential vitamins and proteins removed. However, in the Oriental 7-day reducing diet white rice may be substituted for brown rice (if you cannot get brown rice at your local grocers), for you cannot eat enough of the white rice to put on excess weight. The Chinese, Japanese, and Indonesians, as well as three quarters of the world's population who subsist almost entirely on rice, are notoriously slender and have vitality and energy without having the usual sicknesses of heart disease, high blood pressure, arthritis, and coronary thrombosis.

■ ■ ■

## THE VITAL IMPORTANCE OF THE MEAT PROTEINS

Most people in the Orient cannot afford costly beef, lamb, and pork. They often substitute fish as the main staple to a predominantly rice and vegetable diet. However, as I have stated elsewhere, I have amended the Oriental diet to fit our American needs, where we do have an abundance of protein animal foods in a wide and fairly reasonable assortment.

To the filling Oriental staple of brown rice, one can add the high-protein meats, such as beef, veal, pork, and fish each day, giving a wide variety to the meals as well as assuring that one gets all the vital proteins, without danger of putting on excess weight.

You can usually eat any meat that you desire to give you the day's necessary proteins, and you will find that your body will not turn it into fat.

Now, obviously, you will not want to eat brown rice every day of your life, for this could become monotonous. You can add rice to the diet three or four times a week, and the rest of the time substitute baked or boiled potatoes, which give you carbohydrates and are not fat producing, unless fried or eaten in large quantities.

Besides the high-protein beef, veal, lamb, and pork products, you can add to rice and vegetables the other high-protein foods of poultry, fish, cheese, and eggs. You can get an infinite variety of dishes by using these high-protein foods without risking adding extra weight.

Chuck V. was a 215-pound bulldozer operator. His work was not physically strenuous, although it looked as though it was. He sat eight hours a day and drove the bulldozer, doing no actual physical labor. He was consuming more than 4,000 calories a day, most of it carbohydrates.

At lunchtime Chuck consumed three bread sandwiches, with meat, mayonnaise, or butter, a wedge of fruit pie, and two cups of coffee with sugar and cream. At home he ate meat, bread, potatoes, coffee, usually had a couple of beers while watching TV, and just before going to bed, would have a dish of ice cream and pie or cake, or both. No wonder this man, who was only thirty years of age, was gaining weight and could not seem to stop it.

It was difficult for Chuck to eat the reducing soup and he did not like vegetables, so to get him on a reducing diet was difficult, as he was afraid he would be perpetually hungry and not have enough energy to do his day's work.

In this instance I told Chuck he could eat all the lean meat he desired at lunch, breakfast, and dinner, but he must cut out all bread and butter, pies and cakes, and other sweets. He was to add the brown rice three times a day, with the lean meat, and drink his coffee with artificial sugar and cream, the nondairy kind. In between meals he had been drinking quantities of cokes and soft drinks, with sugar. I told him he could drink the dietetic, sugar-free type of cokes and this would kill his appetite for sweets.

Here is a list of the wide varieties of high-protein meats that are available for your future diet, which assure that you will have variety and highly nutritional protein for the rest of your life, without putting on excess weight, if you eat a normal portion once a day.

■ ■ ■

## HIGH-PROTEIN FOODS YOU CAN SAFELY USE AND HOW TO PREPARE THEM

### Beef

| | |
|---|---|
| chuck and round steak | roast or broil in oven |
| chopped ground steak | broil or fry without fat |
| porterhouse steak | broil |
| T-bone steak | broil |
| tenderloin steak | broil |
| prime ribs of beef | roast |
| sirloin of beef | roast |
| filet mignon | broil |
| short ribs | brown and broil |
| sweetbreads | fry |
| liver | broil or fry without fat |
| kidney | broil |
| heart | stew |
| brains | fry with cooking oil or butter |

### Lamb

| | |
|---|---|
| leg of lamb | roast in oven |
| chopped lamb patties | broil |
| breast of lamb | roast |
| rack of lamb | roast |
| lamb chops | broil |

### Pork

| | |
|---|---|
| fresh ham | boil or roast |
| smoked ham | bake or fry |
| bacon | broil or fry |
| loin of pork | roast |
| spareribs | broil or fry |
| shoulder of pork | bake |
| pork chops | bake or fry |

A word of caution regarding pork products: Even when you are not reducing it is good to limit your consumption of pork to a minimum. It can add taste and variety to your usual routine diet, but all pork products are high in fat, and these are rich foods, high in calories. Now, it is true your body does require some fats, but only about 45 to 60 grams a day, whereas most Americans consume as much as 450 grams of high-calorie fat foods per day. Even a laborer does not need that many fat calories a day.

**Veal**

| | |
|---|---|
| veal cutlets | fry |
| veal steaks | broil |
| round | roast |

**Poultry**

| | |
|---|---|
| chicken | roast, broil, or fry |
| turkey | roast |
| pheasant | roast or broil |
| squab | roast |
| goose (high in fat) | roast |
| duckling (high in fat) | roast |
| guinea hen | roast |

**Fish**

| | |
|---|---|
| halibut | broil or bake |
| salmon, fresh | bake or poach |
| salmon, canned | ready to eat |
| mackerel | broil or bake |
| trout | broil, bake, or fry |
| tuna, canned | ready to eat |
| codfish | broil or bake |
| haddock | broil or bake |
| swordfish | broil, bake, or fry |
| perch | broil, bake, or fry |
| whitefish | bake or broil |
| lobster | broil |
| shrimp | boil or fry |
| crab | boil or fry |
| mussels | steam |
| scallops | broil or fry |
| clams | bake, fry, or raw |
| oysters | bake, fry, or raw |

A word of caution regarding the proteins given above: These are usually to be eaten with caution, even when you are not reducing, for most of them are high in fat content, and they are processed meats that are not as nutritious as fresh meats. They are good to use as luncheon meat in sandwiches or for special occasions, but are not recommended as a steady diet.

### Cheese

Many nutritionists recommend cheese products as good meat substitutes in a diet, but most cheese products are filled with salt and require a great deal of drinking of water. This water is retained in the body cells and often can add as much as ten to fifteen pounds of bloat and weight.

Cheeses should be used sparingly. Cottage cheese, yogurt, and pot cheese are good sources of protein and should be used often.

Whole milk can be used by those who need extra fat in their diets, but most adults can easily use skim milk without the danger of extra fat, and this furnishes valuable proteins and other minerals and vitamins without furnishing the body with extra fat calories that it does not need.

■ ■ ■

## OMELETS AND OTHER EGG DISHES

Eggs can safely be used in most diets as a valuable form of protein, but because of the high cholesterol content of the egg yolk some nutritionists recommend limiting the number of eggs to six a week. But now, with what we know about the healthful side to eggs, more and more doctors are encouraging their patients to consume eggs, as long as the eggs are thoroughly cooked.

### Boiled Eggs

This is a simple way to cook eggs well and safely eat them without fear of bacterial contamination. It's also a very healthful way, since no grease, oil, or butter is required to cook them.

Put eggs into a panful of cold tap water, about 2 cups for 2 eggs, or 4 cups for 6 eggs. Cover the pan and bring the water to a gentle boil. Time the eggs when the water just starts to boil: boiling for about $2^1/_2$ minutes yields a very soft-boiled egg; $7^1/_2$ minutes gives an egg in which the white is solid and the yolk is still a bit soft, and 11 minutes gives a more traditional hard-boiled egg.

Remove the eggs from the water right away with a slotted spoon. Plunge hard-boiled eggs into ice-cold water to make it easier to peel off the shells. By pricking a small hole in the end of each egg with a sewing needle, you will keep older eggs from cracking apart while they're boiling.

### Great Omelets

During the years I worked in the restaurant business I learned from different chefs I trained under that there are a variety of ways to make an omelet. Some cooks I worked with added cream to the eggs, while others used just plain milk. Still others included water or no liquid at all. I once made omelets for a group of vegetarians, and decided to use carrot juice. They raved about the flavor, but when I repeated the same recipe for regular customers later on, they turned their noses up at it, repulsed by the color. For those who like a fruity taste to their omelets, pineapple or orange juice may be substituted for other liquids.

Here is a very basic omelet that can be whipped up in just a few minutes for a light breakfast; it also make an excellent and inexpensive lunch or dinner.

> 2 large grade AA eggs
>
> 2 tsp. water
>
> Pinch of sea salt
>
> 2 tsp. butter for frying pan
>
> *Optional fillings:*
>
>> 2 mushrooms, sliced and lightly sautéed in butter
>>
>> $^1/_4$ cup sliced, cooked chicken
>>
>> 2 Tbsp. well-drained pears

It helps to have a special omelet pan with curving sides to make nicely shaped omelets, but such a pan isn't essential. A fairly heavy nonstick or well-seasoned pan will do, so long as the omelet doesn't stick. But the pan size is important. Too small a pan will yield a thicker-than-usual omelet that isn't cooked all the way through. On the other hand, if the pan is too large, the omelet might end up overcooked before it can be rescued. A 6-inch pan is just the ticket for a two-egg omelet, while an 8-inch pan is nice for a three-egg omelet. Small omelets are much easier to fix than bigger ones.

Heat the pan so that it is medium-hot. Meanwhile, briefly mix the eggs, water, and salt in a small bowl with a fork; a frothy mixture isn't good at all. Remember, you're making an omelet, not scrambled eggs.

Add the butter to the pan. When it foams and begins to brown, pour in the eggs immediately. Cook only for about $2^1/_2$ minutes or until the bottom sets up leaving the top still partially uncooked. Lift up the edges periodically with a spatula to inspect its progress. Your omelet is doing fine if some of the uncooked egg runs down around the edge when you lift up the edges. If you wish to fill the omelet lay the filling ingredient on half of the omelet now. Fold the other half of the omelet over the filling and serve.

One trick that I use to make an omelet look plumper is to lay it on a plate, cover it with a dry paper towel and then, laying my hands on either side of the omelet, gently push them together and tuck some of each side underneath. The idea here is to give it a little more of a circular, oblong shape so it resembles a sausage roll. It also makes the omelet look nicer on the plate as well.

Here are some other tips gleaned from my years in the restaurant business, to help you make great omelets. The eggs should be allowed to sit at room temperature for an hour prior to cooking. Investing in a good, heavy omelet pan is well worth the cost. The pan should be kept seasoned at all times. Never use dish soap in the cleaning process: scrub the pan only with water and salt after each use. Then dry it by heating. While the pan is still hot brush it with some oil on a basting brush. Keep it well oiled for its next use. The pan should always be heated *gradually* until it is good and hot *before* adding the beaten eggs. You can tell when the melted butter is just right for adding the eggs: it will begin making a crackling or sizzling kind of noise at the precise moment they should be poured in.

■ ■ ■

## SOME OMELET FILLINGS

### PERSIAN OMELET

1 Tbsp. butter

$^1/_2$ cup onion, chopped

$^1/_4$ tsp. salt

$^1/_4$ tsp. cumin

$^1/_4$ tsp. cinnamon

$^1/_4$ tsp. turmeric

$^1/_4$ tsp. dry mustard

$^1/_4$ tsp. thyme

Pinches of black pepper and cayenne pepper for flavor

6 large mushrooms, sliced

$^1/_4$ cup slivered, toasted almonds

1 small banana (about 6 inches long), sliced

Parsley, minced

In a medium skillet, sauté the onion in butter, with the salt and all the spices, until the onion is soft (about 6 minutes). Then add the mushroom slices and sauté another 7 minutes. Set aside and stir in the almonds and banana slices. Make the omelet immediately. Put some finely minced parsley into the beaten egg for extra flavor and eye appeal.

### ORIENTAL OMELET

1 large mushroom, cleaned and thinly sliced

2 Tbsp. peanut oil

$^1/_4$ cup drained bamboo shoots, finely chopped

$^1/_4$ cup bean sprouts, finely chopped

3 eggs

Dash of soy sauce

Pinch of granulated kelp

Heat a large, heavy frying pan, about 9 inches in diameter. Sauté the mushroom in oil until lightly browned. Remove it from the pan and temporarily reserve. In the same pan, sauté the bamboo shoots over medium heat, covered, for about 4 minutes, stirring occasionally, until they are lightly browned. Remove them from the pan and set aside. Repeat the same sautéing process with the bean sprouts, but remove the lid to stir every 2 minutes; cook the same way for about 4 minutes as well.

Set the frying pan aside. Break the eggs into a small bowl and add the soy sauce and kelp. Lightly beat them with a fork or a pair of chopsticks. Pour this egg mixture over the sautéed vegetables in the pan; quickly spread them out to distribute them evenly. Return the pan to the heat and cook until the omelet stays together fairly well; allow about 4 minutes for this to happen. Then loosen it from the pan, flip it over on the other side, and cook another $1^1/_2$ minutes. For a little more of an eating challenge, eat the omelet with a pair of chopsticks just like they do in the Orient.

You may want to practice deftly handling a pair of chopsticks before actually using them to eat with. The trick is how you hold them with your fingers and the manipulative action of your wrist.

■ ■ ■

## KEEP VEGETABLES HIGH ON THE LIST OF FOODS TO EAT

With your protein needs adequately provided for in your future diets, do not forget to add a wide variety of vegetables, which are essential to a well-balanced diet. You can now safely include some of the higher-calorie vegetables, which were forbidden when you were on the quick weight-loss diet

You can now expand your list of fresh and cooked vegetables to include the starchier ones such as peas, carrots, and beans. Lima beans are a good staple food, for they not only contain valuable proteins, but have sufficient carbohydrates to satisfy the body's requirements. Navy beans are also excellent for this source—they can be baked, or made into a tasty soup by adding a couple of chopped onions, and a tablespoon of tomato paste.

The following list of vegetables may be consulted for adding variety to your daily intake of these valuable foods.

| | |
|---|---|
| beets | okra |
| carrots | green peppers |
| chard leaves | tomatoes |
| green string beans | eggplant |
| green peas (fresh if possible, | spinach |
| or canned if not) | lettuce |
| corn | watercress |
| kale | broccoli |
| turnips | asparagus |
| mustard greens | brussels sprouts |
| squash | cucumbers |
| artichokes | leeks |
| celery | onions |
| escarole | garlic |
| cabbage | radishes |

■ ■ ■

## WIDE VARIETY OF FRESH FRUITS IN SEASON

To give you the valuable natural sugars for energy, do not neglect the fruits that are in season to give you the balanced nutrition that is so essential to good health. Among these fruits are:

| | |
|---|---|
| apples | watermelon |
| apricots | cantaloupe |
| cherries | oranges |
| strawberries | grapefruit |
| pears | lemons |
| peaches | tangerines |
| grapes | bananas |

The following list of foods represents most of the high-calorie, fattening foods that can be used, although sparingly. You can substitute fruits, figs, dates, and nuts for satisfying the carbohydrate urge that makes people eat so many of the forbidden foods. Avoid these foods in large quantities:

avocado
bacon (unless fat is
    cooked out)
cakes
pies
ice cream
candy (unless it is health
    candy with artificial sugar)
chocolate
coconut
crackers
doughnuts
french dressing or other
    rich dressings (use diet
    dressings only)
all fried foods
gravy
honey

marmalade
syrup
waffles
pancakes
hominy grits
jelly
macaroni
spaghetti
noodles
olive oil
peanut butter
popcorn
potatoes
pretzels
puddings (unless you use the
    sugar-free puddings)
sour cream

■ ■ ■

## USE RAW VEGETABLES WHENEVER POSSIBLE

Most people cook the valuable elements are out of vegetables. The water that is used to cook most vegetables should be saved and used to make gravies (without the addition of fat) or soups. Vegetables are best cooked when slightly steamed, until tender enough to pass a fork through them, with as little water as possible.

But as many raw vegetables as possible should be used as salads. Here are some tasty and nutritious combinations.

Add fresh green lima beans and kernels of corn with raw vegetable salad of lettuce, cucumbers, tomatoes, and green peppers. Use a low-calorie French or Russian dressing.

Make a salad of shredded lettuce, chopped spinach leaves, and watercress. Add tomatoes and cucumbers, and serve with a small portion of cottage cheese or pot cheese, with your favorite salad dressing (the low-calorie variety that can be found on the market shelves or that you can make yourself).

Another good combination is lettuce, chopped celery, spinach leaves, and chopped up tomatoes. Use a dressing of lemon and garlic.

A salad can be made with finely chopped carrots, raw cabbage, and raw beets with greens, finely chopped. Serve with a low-calorie dressing as a luncheon salad with a fish dish.

An avocado salad is high in calories, but if you have been sparing in your fat intake, you can chop up a ripe avocado, celery, green pepper, and onion, and serve on a bed of cut-up lettuce. Use a low-calorie Roquefort or Russian dressing.

■ ■ ■

## SAUCES AND LOW-CALORIE SALAD DRESSINGS TO USE WITH THE ORIENTAL REDUCING DIET

Many times meats and salads can be given taste appeal by using sauces and low-calorie salad dressings that keep you from feeling you are dieting.

Many wonderful sauces can be made by using some of the following ingredients: ketchup, tomato puree, wine or wine vinegar, Worcestershire sauce, and anchovy essence. Use dried herbs, pepper, artificial salt, and other seasonings like garlic powder to add zest to your vegetables, meats, and salads.

### French Dressing

Make enough to fill a large bottle—it will keep indefinitely.

1 cup of tomato juice

$1/4$ tsp. garlic powder

1 cup wine vinegar or tarragon vinegar

$1/2$ tsp. dry mustard

$1/2$ tsp. oregano

A touch of artificial sugar

Artificial salt to taste

A touch of black pepper

Combine the above ingredients in a glass jar and shake thoroughly before using. Store in refrigerator.

## SOUR CREAM SAUCE

2 cups of diet cottage cheese

$1/_2$ tsp. lemon juice

$1/_2$ cup buttermilk

artificial salt

Combine all ingredients. This can be used over fresh vegetable salads, or even fruits.

## HORSERADISH SAUCE

This is good to serve with lean meats or for various types of fish.

Use the sour cream recipe given above and add to this 2 Tbsp. of white or red horseradish.

## SAUCE VINAIGRETTE

2 cloves of garlic, minced or diced

4 Tbsp. water

1 tsp. herbs (tarragon, rosemary, thyme, dill)

$1/_4$ tsp. paprika

Touch of artificial sweetener

Shake together in closed jar and keep in refrigerator.

## CHEESE SAUCE

$1/_2$ cup of buttermilk

$1/_2$ pound farmer cheese

1 egg yolk

$1/_2$ tsp. paprika

2 Tbsp. lemon juice

Salt and pepper to taste

Use a double boiler to prepare this sauce. Melt the cheese in the buttermilk, then put in the egg yolk and blend thoroughly. Add the paprika, salt, pepper, and lemon juice. This is an excellent sauce and can be used over vegetables of all kinds.

### Yogurt Dressing

1 clove of diced garlic

$1/_2$ cup celery leaves

1 tsp. salt

2 Tbsp. tomato paste

2 cups yogurt (plain)

1 cup of diced onions

Artificial sugar

Mix thoroughly in an electric blender until smooth. It is excellent as a dressing for green salads. (Makes about 3 cups.)

### Meat Sauce, Marinade

All lean meats that are intended to be broiled, such as steaks, shishkebab, lamb, and so on, can first be prepared with this marinade sauce and kept wrapped in a plastic bag in the ice box at least overnight. It helps give the meat a delicious flavor.

2 cups of dry red wine

2 tsp. salt

2 tsp. mustard (dry)

2 bay leaves

6 cloves

2 sliced onions

2 cloves garlic, minced

2 stalks celery, chopped

2 cups tarragon vinegar

6 peppercorns

If the above amounts are excessive, store in a glass jar in the refrigerator and use another time.

## Low-Calorie Salad Dressing

3 cups of skim milk

2 tsp. mustard

4 Tbsp. cornstarch

2 egg yolks

$^1/_2$ cup lemon juice

1 tsp. salt substitute

Blend the milk and cornstarch in a double boiler, and heat it until it makes a smooth paste. Mix together the egg yolks, mustard, salts, and lemon juice in a separate bowl. When the milk and cornstarch are a smooth paste over low flame, add the egg mixture to this, until it thickens, and then put into a jar and cool. It can be kept in the refrigerator and used when wanted.

## Tasty French Dressing

2 cups of canned tomato juice

2 Tbsp. cornstarch

4 Tbsp. salad oil

$^1/_2$ cup vinegar

$^1/_2$ tsp. paprika

$^1/_2$ tsp. horseradish

$^1/_2$ tsp. onion salt

$^1/_2$ tsp. celery salt

1 tsp. Worcestershire sauce

$^1/_2$ tsp. dry mustard

$^1/_2$ tsp. garlic powder

Use 1 cup of water in a pan and add cornstarch; stir until it forms a smooth paste. Then add the tomato juice and cook, stirring it, until it is thick. Then cool it and add the other ingredients, beating it until smooth. Store in refrigerator and use as needed.

### BLUE CHEESE DRESSING

1 container of cottage cheese

4 Tbsp. vinegar

4 Tbsp. water

2 8-oz. envelopes of blue cheese salad dressing mix (or you
   may chip up blue cheese or Roquefort chunks if you prefer)

Blend the above ingredients in an electric blender, and store in
a glass jar in the refrigerator. Double the above quantities if you
wish to make up a larger portion to last for longer periods.

### SALAD DRESSING A LA CREME

For this you can use the excellent creamy style salad dressings
found in markets in tinfoil envelopes.

1 cup of tomato juice

4 Tbsp. vinegar

2 envelopes of salad dressing mix

Mix above in a bowl with 4 Tbsp. of water, and store in a glass
jar in the refrigerator.

### HOLLANDAISE SAUCE

2 Tbsp. cream

$1/_2$ tsp. salt

1 Tbsp. vinegar

4 egg yolks

Touch of cayenne pepper

$1/_2$ cup butter

$1/_2$ tsp. dry mustard

pepper to taste

Put a bowl in a pan of hot water and mix egg yolks, vinegar,
cream, salt, and pepper together in a bowl. Put over moderate
heat and beat with an eggbeater. Do not boil water, but let it
become hot. Add butter when the mixture begins to thicken,
beating it until melted.

This sauce is delicious over broccoli, green beans, and asparagus. Also excellent to serve over eggs Benedict.

### YOUR OWN LOW-CALORIE MAYONNAISE

4 egg yolks

2 tsp. salt

$^1/_2$ tsp. paprika

2 tsp. dry mustard

$^1/_2$ tsp. white pepper

$^1/_2$ cup lemon juice

$2^1/_2$ cups salad oil

In a bowl combine the lemon juice, egg yolks, and seasonings. Stir with a rotary beater while adding salad oil slowly, about 1 tablespoon at a time, until all the oil has been used. Add another tablespoon of lemon juice while adding the balance of salad oil, and beat until it is thick. Store in refrigerator.

# HOW TO EXTEND THE 7-DAY ORIENTAL DIET IF YOU WANT TO LOSE MORE THAN TWENTY POUNDS

■ ■ ■

Perhaps you are in the category of people who feel that a weight loss of ten or fifteen pounds is not enough and you want to continue on this Oriental diet to shed from twenty to fifty more pounds safely and without hunger or effort.

You can easily do this by following the basic principles of the Oriental quick weight-loss diet given elsewhere and adding to the diet the combinations and variations that follow. The purpose of this is to give a wide variety of foods to those who are forced to go beyond the one- or two-week periods that most people require to shed only a few pounds. This can be done in a wide variety of ways and by adding low-calorie foods that will keep you perfectly nourished while at the same time melting away the unwanted pounds.

■ ■ ■

## VARIATION DIETS FOR THOSE WANTING TO LOSE MORE THAN TWENTY POUNDS

Many times people want to lose more than twenty pounds, so they have to use the Oriental reducing diet for a period of three or four weeks beyond the seven-day period. The following variation diets may be used to add variety to the diet and also to give more balanced nutrition. The monotony of eating only rice or vegetables, or a combination of these for several weeks, usually discourages people from continuing long enough to shed the additional pounds when they weigh two hundred or more pounds.

### *Woman Lost One Hundred Pounds on the Extended Oriental Diet*

One woman, Mrs. Bernice R., had a difficult weight problem. When she started the Oriental food and diet plan she weighed 250 pounds. She was chronically fatigued, had nervous headaches, high blood pressure, erratic heart action, and was a chronic asthmatic. Her doctors had despaired of her ever losing weight, for she had tried every known diet, all without success. She would lose as much as ten or fifteen pounds and then go off the diet wagon, gaining it right back.

Of course Mrs. R. fell back on the usual excuse when she first came to me out of desperation to help her. "It must be my glands," she moaned as she fell into a large chair. "My mother was heavy all her life. It seems to run in the family, at least on the women's side."

I explained to Mrs. R that usually when the mother is fat, the children also become heavy, owing to the fact that they are all on the same diet, usually a heavy sugar, starch, and carbohydrate diet that sets the eating habits of a youngster early in life. I did not accept the glandular excuse that most people use as a crutch to explain their obesity.

Mrs. R. began with the two-day fasting period, and immediately had high hopes when she saw she had lost 5 pounds. Of course, this was excess water she had accumulated in her tissues, but it gave her courage to continue the Oriental diet.

After two weeks on the stringent diet of only vegetables and brown rice, she had shed another 25 pounds, but she was terribly tired of the monotony of being denied other foods. It was then that she went on the extended variation diets, for I could see she would have to vary the diet if she was to remain on it and shed another 70 pounds. I estimated that she could easily get rid of about 10 pounds a week, which would take her seven more weeks of sticking with the diet.

I put her on a vegetable-and-meat diet for the third week of the diet, and she registered 12 pounds less at the end of the week.

The next week she went on the fish-and-tomato diet, which allowed her to eat any kind of fish, such as bass, tuna, salmon, shrimp, lobster, halibut, abalone, or flounder, broiled, and two medium-sized tomatoes at each meal. She could eat tomatoes between meals also.

Then Mrs. R. started the lean-meat-and-tomato regimen for the next week, and again showed a loss of 12 pounds.

The next week she ate all the vegetables she wanted from the list that follows, which gave her three or four vegetables a day, and as these were the reducing vegetables, she was able to continue losing even when she stuffed herself.

For one full week she went on the low-calorie reducing fruits, eating all she wanted of watermelon, cantaloupe, apples, and pumpkin. In that one week she was able to rid herself of 15 more pounds. The reason for the quicker weight loss on fruits was that these fruits all require more calories to digest than they give to the body. Naturally, she could not continue on such a stringent diet indefinitely without harm to her health, but for only one week it did no harm. She drank eight to ten glasses of water a day, and as the body was not receiving any fat whatsoever on this diet, it was being forced to burn up its own fat! This is one reason why she was able to lose the 100 pounds in such a short time. As she had to have some other variations to the diet for such a long period of time, she began to eat some boiled eggs, or cottage cheese with her fruits and vegetables, and also skim milk—two glasses a day fortified with two tablespoons of powdered dry milk.

I observed Mrs. R. over a period of many months after she had completed her strenuous reducing and am happy to report that periodic checkups with her personal doctor while she dieted and afterward revealed that many of her physical symptoms began to disappear with the fat. Today, she is down to her desired weight of about 150 pounds.

■ ■ ■

## FISH-AND-TOMATO DIET

For one entire week, during four weeks or more of the Oriental diet, use the fish-and-tomato-only plan. Each day you may eat half a pound of delicious broiled fish. This can be eaten three times a day! You need not worry about putting on too many calories on this diet, and it is excellent for fish lovers. In other words, you are actually eating one and a half pounds of fish on this diet, enough to more than satisfy your protein needs. You do not add any carbohydrates, sugars or starches. You do not add vegetables, or even rice on this variation plan. During that week you will probably tire of this fish diet, and then want to go on to another of our variation Oriental diets, where you can still continue to lose five to seven pounds a week until the desired weight has been achieved.

You may select any of the following types of fish:

| | |
|---|---|
| tuna (canned or fresh) | flounder |
| sea bass | halibut |
| cod steaks | salmon |
| shrimp | abalone |
| lobster | shad roe |
| oysters | |

You can use three varieties of fish on any one day, which will give you a wide variety without tiring your taste buds. For breakfast you can use creamed tuna on a piece of whole-wheat toast rather than cereal or eggs. It is an excellent protein substitute and will not endanger the calorie intake.

■ ■ ■

## THE SECOND WEEK YOU MIGHT TRY MEAT AND TOMATOES ONLY

I have personally seen many people drop pounds of excess weight using only meat and tomatoes. You can eat half a pound of any lean meat three times a day, which gives a total intake of one and a half pounds of this protein food. Drink plenty of water on this meat-and-tomatoes diet, for it helps flush out all the excess acid ash and uric acid that a great deal of meat gives the body. You can eat three tomatoes a day, raw or canned, and this diet will give you a perpetually full feeling without that strong craving most dieters have for starches and sugars.

Some of the low-calorie meats you may use on this diet are

filet mignon
ground lean meat (broiled or fried without fat)
liver (broiled)
T-bone steak
sirloin steak
tenderloin steak
lamb chops or breast of lamb
veal
pork chops (broiled, with fat removed)
pot roast
sweetbreads

A good variation on breakfast while you are on your meat-and-tomato diet is to have broiled kidneys on toast, or sweetbreads on toast, or chipped beef on whole-wheat toast.

This meat-and-tomato diet is a rich variation to the usual reducing plans given in this book, but is not to be encouraged as a steady diet, for it is essential that vegetables, fruits, some carbohydrates, and fats be added to the regular sustaining diets. It must be used only as a means for breaking up the monotony of the usual reducing diets.

■ ■ ■

## ALL-VEGETABLE DIET

A wonderful variation to the regular Oriental 7-day diet for one week is an all-vegetable diet, which gives you a large choice of vegetables that will never add weight but will furnish you with most of the body's nutritive elements.

Certain vegetables are higher in calories than others and should be avoided for the one-week vegetable diet. The forbidden vegetables are

avocados
beans (white)
lentils
sweet potatoes
corn

You can eat several meals of just vegetables, as many as six meals a day, without worrying about eating too many calories. In fact, some people who choose to be vegetarians live on nothing but vegetables, with some milk products, eggs, nuts, and grains, and occasionally fish. They never eat red-blooded meat of any kind, and these people remain remarkably slender and seem to have tremendous energy and vitality. However, I do not recommend a complete vegetarian diet unless you have carefully checked with your doctor to see that there are not special conditions in your case that require greater variation in your food intake.

You may select from a wide variety of vegetables from the following list and vary them from day to day, eating as much as you want for each meal. Your capacity is limited when it comes to vegetables, so it becomes impossible to overeat. The following vegetables furnish the body with fewer calories that others, and require more calories to digest than they give to the body.

| | | |
|---|---|---|
| tomatoes | broccoli | mushrooms |
| turnips | cabbage | sauerkraut |
| lettuce | brussels sprouts | cauliflower |
| green peppers | celery | leeks |
| radishes | asparagus | kohlrabi |
| cucumbers | string beans | garlic |
| watercress | spinach | okra |

The following vegetables may be added if your continue the vegetable diet beyond the first week, although these have more fat calories than vegetables in the previous list.

| | |
|---|---|
| beets | squash |
| carrots | rutabagas |
| kale | parsnips |
| onions | chives |
| red peppers | artichokes |

You can steam the vegetables until they are soft, and then to add some flavor you may use a little melted butter. The fat calories from this flavoring are allowed, as there are no other forms of fat or starch in this diet.

You can eat as many varieties of vegetables each day as you wish, using about one cup of each per day. You might select several vegetables one day and others the next day, giving a variety so you do not tire of them. You could eat as many as fifteen cups of these vegetables a day, in addition to a large fresh tomato and a head of lettuce, with a low-calorie dressing, and you would hardly exceed 900 calories per day.

However, if you begin to add other foods and use high-calorie dressings on the raw vegetable salads, you soon will have several hundred more calories, which will be fat calories that put your weight back on quickly.

You can use herbs, spices, and low-calorie dressings to give taste and variety to your vegetables. You can also eat a large baked potato with butter for the evening meal, but you should avoid all eggs, cheese, cream, bread, nuts, milk, and other foods that would tend to unbalance this vegetable diet.

However, if you should decide to choose the lactovegetarian diet as a sustaining diet for the remainder of your life, you may safely add some butter; cheese, including cottage cheese and pot cheese; yogurt; nuts; grains; and rice, and you can be assured that you will never again have a weight problem. This natural diet of natural foods is the nearest thing to our pure Oriental food plan, for remember, most people in the Eastern countries cannot eat meat, as it is prohibitively expensive, and many are forbidden to eat the flesh of animals by their religions, so they exist entirely on the lactovegetarian foods given above.

You may achieve more rapid weight loss on an all-fruit diet than on the all-vegetable diet, and it is much more palatable to your taste buds, as well as highly nutritious. You can start your fruit diet with breakfast, then eat at least six or seven times a day, and never fear that you are overdoing.

There are two categories of fruits that you may use in the all-fruit reducing plan. The first one includes those fruits that require more calories to digest than they give to the body. The ones on the other list add some calories. These two groups may be intermingled, so select some fruits from the first list and add a few from the second list.

However, if your aim is a complete loss of several pounds you should stick to those low-calorie fruits given in list number one.

### List No. 1—The Low-Calorie Reducing Fruits

cantaloupe
pumpkin
honeydew melon
watermelon
rhubarb

### List No. 2—The Higher-Calorie Fruits

| | | |
|---|---|---|
| peaches | apples | oranges |
| pears | cherries | cranberries |
| blackberries | grapes | nectarines |
| apricots | grapefruit | papaya |
| lemons | pineapples | raspberries |
| limes | plums | fresh strawberries |
| loganberries | prunes (fresh) | tangerines |

Should you eat canned fruits on this all-fruit diet? Only if fresh fruits are not available or in season. Then you should select brands that are packed in low-calorie, sugar-free syrup, found on the shelves of dietetic foods in your grocery store. If you use regular canned fruits in heavy syrup be sure to wash off the syrup.

If you wish to continue your all-fruit diet into the second or third weeks, and you continue to lose from five to ten pounds a week, you may add interesting variations, such as cottage cheese, boiled eggs, vegetables, yogurt, and skim milk.

You may also use a variation that many people like, as it continues to help them lose weight, while at the same time satisfying their taste buds with a delicious variety. This is a combination of fruits and vegetables taken from this above lists. Mix two or more vegetables and fruits from the above lists, and eat at least four or five times a day, or whenever you are hungry. You need not bother counting calories in this diet, for you can seldom eat more than 900 or 1000 calories a day on this fruit-and-vegetable diet. After consuming a few cupfuls of fruits and vegetables you will have a comfortably full feeling. Then add several glasses of water per day, at least eight, and you will never have that hungry, gnawing feeling that comes when you are on the usual diet.

Bananas are not given in the above lists of fruits for an obvious reason—they are highly placed in the carbohydrate list of foods. However, if you have a craving for bananas, you can try a banana and skim milk diet for one week, and you will find you will still continue to lose weight and at the same time indulge your craving for starches and carbohydrates. Each banana contains about 85 calories, and skim milk per glass is about 90 calories. You can alternate your bananas and skim milk, and eat as many as eight good-sized bananas and eight glasses of skim milk a day, and not consume more than 900 to 1000 calories a day.

### *Bananas and Skim Milk Rid Him of Twenty-Five Unwanted Pounds*

Burt E. weighed 210 pounds when he started his Oriental reducing diet, and he kept at it faithfully for the first two weeks, getting rid of 15 pounds a week. But then he got tired of the monotony of the diet, so I suggested he try the bananas-and-skim-milk diet, eating about eight bananas a day and drinking at least eight glasses of skim milk per day. This was a pleasant variety to his diet, as he liked bananas, and he was able to keep this up for one week, without monotony. He lost only 10 pounds that week, but as he now weighed 170 pounds, which was about normal for him, he went on the sustaining diet and kept his weight at that level in the months I observed him. He was an office worker, and it was no great difficulty for him to reduce his caloric intake to less than 1000 calories during the several weeks he needed to shed his weight.

■ ■ ■

## ALTERNATING DIETS

You might try alternating your fruit, vegetable, and banana days as follows:

One day use the all-fruit diet
The second day use the all-vegetable diet
The third day try using the vegetable-and-fruit diet
The fourth day use the milk-and-banana diet
The fifth day you might use the meat-only diet
The sixth day you can use the meat-and-vegetable diet
The seventh day use brown rice and vegetables

Another interesting variation to our Oriental 7-day diet is based on milk and milk products. You can use this for a one-week variation, and you can be sure that you will continue to lose pounds while at the same time satisfying your taste buds.

On any given day you can use fruit-flavored yogurt to add variety. You can use cottage cheese or pot cheese for lunch, with a piece of fruit, such as a pear or peach. For dinner you can eat a cheese omelet, made with two eggs, and fried without fat.

Each day you can drink as many as six glasses of skim milk, starting at breakfast, and fortify the skim milk with powdered milk. This gives added proteins and more energy.

You may drink buttermilk one day, to add variety. You can also vary this diet by eating other milk products, such as cheddar or other cheese. Cheese should be used carefully, however, as it is a high-calorie food. Only a two-inch square should be consumed in a day while on this cheese-and-milk diet plan.

■ ■ ■

## BROWN-RICE-AND-EGG REDUCING PLAN

I have seen many people lose weight quickly on a brown-rice-and-egg diet for one week, which they used to add variety to the above plans.

You can poach or fry an egg and serve it on top of the rice, with a little melted butter, and this can be eaten as often as three or four times a day. Breakfast can include eight ounces of orange juice or other fruit juice, one slice of whole-wheat toast, and the egg-and-rice combination.

You can also vary this egg diet for the week by having, every other day, an egg omelet—one time use cheese for filler, the next time use mushrooms, another time use chips of bacon (out of which all the fat has been removed by frying). Green peppers and onions can be added for another meal. With the omelets you can serve a small portion of rice.

# CHAPTER 13

# How to Use the Oriental Diet Plan to Give You Added Joy in Love and Sex

■ ■ ■

## THE ORIENTAL DIET PLAN ADDS TO LIFE'S JOYS

One reason why the Oriental diet plan can improve your sexual vigor and give you a more romantic outlook on life is the fact that you will be taking more vitalized, live foods into your body than you were formerly. You will also be able to eat more frequently, at least six times a day, of the vitalizing and yet reducing foods, so that your body receives a constant flow of energy without making you feel sluggish, nervous, and exhausted.

A study on physical efficiency and sexual vitality was made at a famous Eastern university. A startling fact was discovered: When a person ate only three regular meals a day, he stuffed his system with many unnecessary foods that lacked nutritive value and affected his energy and sexual potency. When the meals were reduced in size and the person ate six times a day, it was discovered that he gained vitality, felt less nervous and irritable, and had a stronger sexual drive.

What is the reason for this difference? As the body requires certain amino acids, found mostly in protein foods, to function properly, it was found that in three meals a day there was less chance that all of the twenty-two different amino acids would be taken into the body. But if the meals are increased to six a day, as we suggest in our Oriental system of dieting, there is a good chance that most of these amino acids will be ingested.

The foods that are richest in these essential elements are meat, fish, cheese, soybeans, and rice in its unprocessed, natural state, where the protein is left in the husk.

In our balanced reducing diet, and also in the sustaining diet after losing your necessary pounds, you will continue to receive these highly important amino acids that give you feelings of well-being and that increase sexual vigor and potency.

Scientists established a long time ago that the body requires eight particular amino acids so it can survive—these are the *essential* amino acids. Beyond them, however, are other nonessential amino acids, which the body isn't necessarily dependent upon for staying alive. But these nonessential ones also serve important purposes, too, in their own way.

Tyrosine is one such nonessential amino acid. The tyrosine content of white matter within the brain is small and only minimally concentrated in the cerebrospinal fluid of the spinal cord. But this is just enough to serve as a precursor for certain hormones responsible for sexual stimulation. When taken in the form of L-tyrosine, this nonessential amino acid is very helpful in increasing sexual drive in men and women. By increasing dietary tyrosine, doctors specializing in the treatment of sexual dysfunction have found that dopamine concentrations in the brain are raised; by doing so, sexual drive is remarkably enhanced.

A good friend of mine, a doctor from New Jersey who treats many older sexually crippled people, told me about a particular case he treated a while back. A seventy-three-year-old man came to his clinic with a decade-long history of reduced sex drive almost to the point of impotence. An interview revealed that the patient was quite intense in most of his mannerisms. Surprisingly though, a check of his blood pressure showed it to be somewhat on the low side. He was placed on one-half gram of tyrosine at 8:30 A.M. and the same amount again at 5:30 P.M. Two weeks later this amount was doubled to one gram in the morning and the same intake repeated in the evening. Within six weeks his sex drive had returned, much to his own amazement and the delight of his wife.

L-tyrosine has been used by nutritional-minded doctors to treat depression, low self-esteem, anxiety, frustration, food allergies, and migraines in many of their overweight patients. They've discovered that it is a wonderful mood elevator. Better news still is that L-tyrosine is a great appetite suppressant. But, best of all, regular intake of this nonessential amino acid (in its free form) helps to reduce body fat.

There are several ways of getting more L-tyrosine into your system. One, of course, is through regular supplementation. Between two and four capsules or tablets daily have been recommended by many therapists. They also encourage their patients to take a high-potency B complex along with the L-tyrosine: one vitamin B tablet for every two L-tyrosine capsules/tablets, or two vitamin B tablets for every four of the other. Figure on taking 1,000 milligrams of L-tyrosine daily in divided doses.

L-tyrosine can also be produced from L-phenylalanine. The artificial sweetener known as aspartame contains a great deal of phenylalanine; when it is taken into the body in the form of NutraSweet (its commercial name), tyrosine concentrations in the brain are dramatically increased. This always seems to be beneficial for increasing sexual drive. *Note:* If you are allergic to aspartame, you should *not* be using NutraSweet or anything else containing aspartame.)

You won't find much tyrosine in fruits, vegetables, and plant oils, and hardly any is to be found in cereals and grains. But certain other foods are reasonably high in tyrosine content. By including them more frequently in your diet, you can certainly help your sex drive. The table that follows shows which foods can be used for this.

| Food | Amount | Gram Content |
|------|--------|--------------|
| Wild game | 1 lb. | 3 |
| Chinese suckling pig (or regular pork) | 1 lb. | 2.5 |
| Cottage cheese | 1 cup | 1.7 |
| Ricotta cheese | 1 cup | 1.5 |
| Turkey | 1 lb. | 1.3 |
| Beijing duck | 1 lb. | 1.1 |
| Rex's Wheat Germ Oil* | 1 cup | 1 |

*You may obtain Rex's Wheat Germ Oil (1-quart can) by sending $65 to: Anthropological Research Center, POB 11471, Salt Lake City, UT 84147.

Other nutrients that are helpful for increasing sex drive in older individuals are: zinc, 75 mg.; vitamin A, 25,000 I.U.; vitamin C, 3,500 mg.; papaya tablet, one per meal. And herbs such as yohimbine, Korean ginseng, and ginkgo biloba are all equally effective, too, in revving up sexual drive that has been parked for years in one spot. The average intake of any of these herbs, either separately or in combination with one another, is two capsules of each daily. Bee pollen and royal jelly are also useful as well.

■ ■ ■

## FOODS THAT ADD TO SEXUAL POTENCY AND VITALITY

The following foods are high in amino acids and in lecithin, the food supplement that helps in reducing the cholesterol level in the bloodstream. As lecithin has been found to play a vital role in the life function of the living cells, it is thought to be an essential element in maintaining the body's sexual vigor at a high level into advanced old age.

Amino acids are found plentifully in the following foods:

Lean beef, lamb, pork, and veal
Soybeans, soybean oil, soybean flour, soybean powder
Fish
Cheese
Beans—navy and lima, as well as lentils (also have some proteins)

Brown rice has some of these essential proteins and amino acids. This is one reason why it is a valuable basic food in any diet, to be eaten at least three or four times a week when on the sustaining diet.

Lecithin is found plentifully in soybean powder and oil (which can be added to cereals for breakfast, or to salads or soups). It is also prominent in certain seeds that can be munched between meals. These include sunflower, pumpkin, and sesame seeds. In fact, these seeds contain even more lecithin than soybeans! They should be eaten daily if one wants sexual vigor and a high degree of vitality and energy.

Mr. T. L. was a man of sixty when I first met him through my lecture work in New York City. He was 30 pounds overweight, weighing 195 pounds when he should have weighed 165 pounds for his age and height. But being overweight was not his only problem. In our first interview he told me he had been sexually impotent for three years, and his wife had accepted the fact that this was probably due to the aging process. She was five years younger than he, and still had sexual desires, which she now had to suppress.

Before he began the Oriental system of reducing, I had him check carefully with his doctor, who gave him the go-ahead signal, as he was in fairly good condition physically. He had slight symptoms of high blood pressure, which varied from time to time. He was a heavy smoker and drank coffee all day long to keep up his energy for his work.

T. L. responded to the Oriental diet beautifully, and the first week he was able to lose 12 pounds. This encouraged him, so he kept at the diet, with variations, until in two months' time he had completely shed the 30 unwanted pounds!

But changing his dietary habits was also necessary if he was to overcome his problem of sexual impotence.

I remembered a guru I had once met in India who was more than a hundred years of age, and he told me about the wonders of soybean oil, which is high in lecithin. He also told me about sunflower and pumpkin seeds, which he munched on all day between meals. He claimed that these foods contain natural elements that would prolong sexual vigor into the eighties.

I told T. L. about soybean oil, and also about the sunflower and pumpkin seeds, suggesting that he might try them to increase his sexual potency.

I did not hear anything further from T. L. for a month, and I had completely forgotten him when one day my telephone rang, and a vigorous, joyous voice on the other end proclaimed, "Well, Doc, your soybean oil and seeds worked miracles! For the first time in several years I am like a young man of thirty! My wife and I are going on our second honeymoon. We're like a couple of kids in love for the first time!"

Since that time I have seen amazing results from the therapy of soy bean oil, soybean flour, and soybean powder, as well as from sunflower, pumpkin, and sesame seeds, all of which are rich in lecithin. This should be something that is added to all normal diets, not just on the reducing diet, since it gives the body many important amino acids and other elements that are essential to the maintenance of good health.

Wheat germ, as well as natural, unprocessed barley, oats, and buckwheat, contains vital elements that also give vitality and energy when used in their natural state.

■ ■ ■

## THE IMPORTANCE OF YOUR THYROID GLAND

One of the most important glands that determines how young you remain, and whether you retain or lose your sexual vigor, is the thyroid gland, which is located in the throat. This gland affects the metabolic rate of the body—if it is too active in its secretion of thyroxin, you will be in a state of constant nervous activity, you will be restless, and you will suffer from insomnia and other symptoms; if it secretes too slowly, you find you seldom have enough energy to keep you going through the day, and you may drink cups of coffee or smoke dozens of cigarettes to give you the energy boost you feel you need.

One of the vital elements that will keep your body in good health and give you youthful sexual vigor throughout life is iodine. In fact, the thyroid requires iodine to keep it functioning perfectly. It is true that only small amounts of iodine are needed, and these should be from natural foods. (The iodine used for medication on wounds is *not* the type to be used in the diet.) Iodine is found plentifully in fish and also in garlic. Iodized salt is also a good source for obtaining the small amounts one needs, if one eats salt. Some people eat sea salt, which is sold in health food stores and this is also a good source of this vital element. There is also a form of dried kelp or seaweed that can be used for obtaining iodine in the diet.

When the thyroid gland malfunctions it has very serious repercussions on the health, affecting the sex glands especially. They become sluggish and sometimes inactive, making a person unable to respond to a sexual stimulus. Adequate amounts of iron combined with iodine in the diet, have tremendous power to implement the sex drive and affects the heart, brain, endocrine system, and blood vessels, giving an impetus to all these and making a person sexually vigorous and healthy for old age.

■ ■ ■

## SEX POWER DEPENDS ON THE MINERALS IN THE DIET

Even when you are on the Oriental reducing diet, keep in mind that your body must continue to be supplied with the minerals and other elements necessary to good nourishment and to keep the body functioning at high levels of energy.

Iron in the blood not only gives that extra boost to sex energy and general vitality, but it is essential to keep the nails, hair, muscles, bones, and teeth in good condition. Also, iron is helpful in maintaining the balance between the body's alkalinity and acidity, which can affect the body's chemistry. When mineral intake is insufficient, the health suffers, for iron affects the nerves that send messages to the entire body for its proper functioning. Iron also helps the body assimilate many nutrients required for maintaining perfect health and sexual vigor.

Elsewhere we have discussed the minerals that can be taken in supplements to a diet, if you do not obtain them through natural foods. These necessary minerals are

iron
phosphorous
calcium
copper
manganese
potassium
sodium

## Iron

Iron is found in its natural state in all green leafy vegetables; also in soybeans, wheat germ, egg yolk, liver, and bran. Blackstrap molasses is also a good source of iron.

## Phosphorus

Phosphorus can be obtained in its natural state in most protein foods, such as fish, meats, cheese, poultry, eggs, whole-wheat products, and soybeans.

If you do not want to take these minerals in supplements you can take them in foods, but it is easier to be sure you obtain the right amounts by taking one or two vitamin supplements a day; or, consult your doctor regarding your exact needs if you have a special condition that needs treatment.

## Calcium

If you are getting plenty of calcium in your daily diet but eat a great deal of white bread, chocolate, or absorb the chemical DDT from unwashed vegetables or fruits, you may be inhibiting the absorption of this vital element. Calcium is to be found most plentifully in milk, egg yolk, olives, most cheese products, blackstrap molasses, green vegetables, seafood, poultry, and whole grains.

## Copper

When there is a deficiency in this vital mineral a person is apt to have anemia, for copper and iron work together to help enrich the blood. Also, copper plays a part in pigment formation and a lack of it can often cause prematurely gray hair.

Copper is to be found in oatmeal, leafy greens, liver, soybeans, wheat germ, blackstrap molasses, bran, and egg yolk. Huckleberries are also rich in this mineral.

## Manganese

It is claimed that an absence of this mineral in the daily diet can lead to a lessening of interest in sexual expression. A lack often has been found to interfere with normal functioning of the reproductive glands. As manganese works with calcium and phosphorous, it helps activate a number of the body's enzymes. You find little of this vital mineral in the refined foods, but it is to be found in cereals, green vegetables, and whole grains. Wheat germ sprinkled over salads or used in breakfast cereals is a good source of this mineral.

### Potassium

Potassium is often cooked out of vegetables when they are overcooked. It is best to steam vegetables until you can pass a fork through them, not to cook them until they fall apart.

This vital mineral helps the nerves, the heart, and muscles, and gives tone and nourishment. When it is lacking in the diet a person may feel irritable, suffer from indigestion, and be constipated. Those who suffer from insomnia often lack potassium their diets.

Potassium is to be found in green leafy vegetables, sea kelp, cranberries, tomatoes, apple cider vinegar, blackstrap molasses, cucumbers, carrots, and honey. Many fruits also contain this vital mineral.

### Sodium

This important mineral is often thought to exist in salt, but it does not, for salt is sodium chloride and does not supply the necessary sodium to the diet. It can be obtained from green string beans, celery, zucchini, and many other vegetables.

In using the Oriental system of dieting, and the sustaining diet after losing weight, keep in mind always that if you want your body to maintain its youthful vigor and sexual potency until old age, you cannot be twenty to thirty pounds overweight. There is a marked drop in energy when you carry fat around, and it naturally affects your joy in living, as well as your sexual expression and feelings.

I remember carrying a twenty-pound turkey home from the market one holiday. Although it was only two blocks to my house, when I got there I felt exhausted! I thought then that if a person carrying twenty pounds of excess fat twenty-four hours a day felt the same way, no wonder he could not perform his life's functions and his work efficiently and with joy. Fat robs us of the joy of living, not only in reduced sexual desires but in every other department of our lives.

When you get the weight off with the Oriental reducing system, you can keep it off by following the sensible rules given in this chapter.

# How to Satisfy Your Sweet Tooth on the Oriental Reducing Diet Without Adding Weight

■ ■ ■

**W**hile you are on our Oriental diet for losing weight without hunger, you can still eat many wonderful desserts and be safely within your caloric requirements for the day, without the fear of adding weight.

How do the Orientals satisfy their cravings for sweets? Fortunately for them, they cannot afford the rich starches, sugars, and carbohydrates that we eat in this country, and are forced to rely on the natural fruits, dates, figs, honey, and other products that are indigenous to their countries.

■ ■ ■

## FRESH-FRUIT DESSERTS

Following is a list of the fresh fruits that may be used in season for preparing some of the desserts that will give your sweet tooth satisfaction without adding extra weight.

| | |
|---|---|
| apples | mangoes |
| apricots | nectarines |
| bananas | oranges |
| blueberries | papayas |
| blackberries | peaches |
| cantaloupe | pears |
| cherries | persimmons |
| currants | pineapple (fresh or canned) |
| gooseberries | plums |
| grapefruit | raspberries |
| grapes | rhubarb |
| guavas | strawberries |
| honeydew melon | tangerines |
| loganberries | watermelon |

Remember, while on the Oriental 7-day diet to lose weight, you do not need to deny your craving for sweets. But it is important to know that you can add the following desserts to your regular diet only by eating smaller portions than if you were not dieting. Any food, even meat, if excessively eaten, adds many unnecessary calories and is converted into fat. This is why later I shall give you calorie counting as an adjunct to your sustaining diet, so that you will become accustomed to thinking in terms of your required calories and not go overboard on any of the foods you eat in the future.

For some of the exotic desserts given, you can use a pie crust made the health food way, with whole-wheat flour, and by blending the following ingredients. This will keep in your freezer indefinitely, and it may be used as a base for many desserts made with fresh or canned fruits. You will need:

2 cups of whole-wheat flour

1 cup of sour cream

$1/_2$ tsp. salt

1 tsp. of brown sugar

1 cake of yeast

$1/_4$ pound of butter

Blend the brown sugar and the yeast with the sour cream until it is a thick paste, and then let the mixture rise for about an hour.

Use sea salt rather than regular salt and mix this with the butter. Add the sour cream mixture, and knead in a bowl. Add more flour if you find the dough sticks in the pan or seems to be too soft, until it is easy to handle. Now roll the dough into a thin pie crust and line the bottom of a pie plate when you want to add the various fruits we shall give for desserts.

### HIMALAYAN APRICOT TARTS

Cut in halves a pound of fresh, ripe apricots, place these on the crust just described, and cut into smaller portions in individual small tin dishes. Or, if you choose to make an entire pie, use a pie tin and spread the dough over it, putting in the filler of fruits and other ingredients.

Top the apricots with yogurt blended with a tablespoon of honey.

Put into the oven and bake for 30 minutes at about 340°F.

### TIBETAN SNOWMAN DESSERT

Use lemon or orange sherbet, or if you choose, raspberry sherbet. Sprinkle coconut (shredded) on top, and before serving add a spoonful of grenadine or real rum.

This is a dessert that is low in calories and yet gives the impression of being a real sweet dessert.

### PAPAYA SHANGRI-LA

This delicious fruit has many vitamins and minerals that are excellent for any diet, reducing or sustaining. You can cut a papaya in half and stuff the halves with chopped prunes, nuts, and a little honey, topped with yogurt. It is rich and flavorful and satisfies the appetite after a light meal, or it may be eaten as a salad at lunch with a slice of date-nut bread.

### BOMBAY BANANA BANQUET

2 sliced bananas

2 tsp. lemon juice

2 egg whites, unbeaten

Sea salt

1 spoonful honey

1 tsp. vanilla

Nutmeg or cinnamon

Thoroughly mix the banana and the lemon juice by mashing them together, then add the egg white, a touch of sea salt, and the spoonful of honey and vanilla. Blend all these together in your electric blender until they are thoroughly mixed.

Put into four sherbet glasses and top with a touch of cinnamon or nutmeg.

This adds a festive touch to your lunch or dinner, and if you have guests they will think it is a rich dessert, and they will not even know that you are on a diet. The bananas are carbohydrates, of course, but you need some carbohydrates each day, so let this dessert furnish it for this day.

### SULTAN'S HAREM AMBROSIA

This dessert may be served in sherbet glasses, either hot or cold. It is slightly stimulating to the emotions, as one of the ingredients is dry red wine. It is good after a light dinner and gives the impression of being a rich dessert, and yet it has few calories. You need:

4 Tbsp. honey

4 egg yolks

4 Tbsp. dry red wine

Beat these together until thoroughly blended, and then put them into a pan and apply medium heat until the mixture begins to boil, then turn off the heat. Be sure to keep beating the mixture constantly while cooking, until it is thickened and quite fluffy. Put into sherbet dishes and cool, or serve hot.

## Cleopatra's Slimming Nectar

To satisfy your taste buds during your 7-day Oriental reducing diet, you can take this delicious fruit drink two or three times a day, between your normal six meals. It will give you valuable minerals and other elements, without adding weight.

Mix together equal parts of cranberry juice, pineapple juice, and apricot juice, and add the juice of half a lemon. Serve after cooling in the refrigerator.

## Cashmere Honey Pears

For this dessert you can use canned pears if fresh pears are not available. Be sure to wash off the syrup or use pears that are dietetically canned, with a sugar substitute. Drain off the juice. Then assemble the following:

8 pear halves

1 Tbsp. honey

1 Tbsp. lemon juice

1 tsp. cinnamon

2 Tbsp. butter

Sour cream

Place the pear halves in a buttered dish, pour the lemon and honey over the pears, and sprinkle with cinnamon, with small pieces of butter on top. Bake in oven heated to 350°F for about 15 minutes or less, and serve with cold sour cream on top.

### Baghdad Custard Rice Pudding

| | |
|---|---|
| $1/2$ cup brown rice | 4 cups milk |
| $1/4$ cup brown sugar | 4 Tbsp. cold water |
| 2 Tbsp. plain gelatin | 1 tsp. vanilla |
| 1 tsp. almond extract | 1 cup whipped cream (artificial) |

Cook the rice in a double boiler until it is tender, usually about an hour. Be sure to stir it occasionally to keep it from sticking to the pan. Soak gelatin and sugar in the cold water for about 4 minutes. Then add them to the rice. Let this stand until cold, and then stir in the vanilla and almond extracts. Put in the refrigerator to chill until ready to serve, then top it with the artificial whipped cream.

### Bananas a la Nirvana

Bananas are an excellent source of carbohydrates and should be used frequently in desserts.

This celestial delight is easy to make and very delicious. You will need:

6 or 7 bananas

3 Tbsp. brown sugar or honey

$1/2$ tsp. cinnamon

1 tsp. ground ginger

3 Tbsp. butter

$1/2$ lb. cream cheese

1 cup plain yogurt

Brown the halved bananas slightly in butter. Then put 6 halves into a slightly buttered pie plate. Mix the brown sugar or honey with the cream cheese and the cinnamon, and spread half of the mixture over the 6 banana halves. Then put the remaining bananas on top and spread the balance of the mixture. Top with the yogurt and place in oven for 20 minutes at about 350°F. Serves 6.

### KASHMIR APRICOT DELIGHT

The apricot is a very valuable food, and many people of the Middle East and Far East use them as a dietary staple, either fresh or dried. You can use dried apricots for this delicious dessert, soaking them in cold water overnight until soft. You will need:

8 to 10 whole apricots

6 egg whites, beaten until stiff

$1/4$ tsp. artificial salt

5 Tbsp. honey or brown sugar

$1/4$ tsp. almond extract

Shred the apricots in a beater until they become pulp. Be sure the eggs are beaten until firm, then put the apricots into the beaten eggs with all the other ingredients. Put into a greased double boiler and cook for an hour.

You can serve this apricot delight with pineapple or grape juice as a sauce. Or you can top it with artificial whipped cream, or a spoonful or sour cream or yogurt.

### INDIAN PRINCESS ORANGE TEMPTATION

This simple and yet nutritious and healthful dessert is made with just oranges and shredded coconut, and yet it gives an exotic look to your after-dinner dessert if you have guests. All you need are

5 oranges, (thinly sliced)

$2/3$ cup of shredded coconut

On top of a layer of sliced oranges, sprinkle coconut, then continue the process, with a layer of oranges, again topped with the shredded coconut. Sprinkle chopped nuts on top and chill.

A wide variety of fruit cups can be used for desserts. They will add variety to your meals and give the impression you are having something sweet at the end of your meal, yet the calories contained in these various fruit cups are few.

You can combine pears and apricots, using canned pears, and canned apricots. Combine these in a compote dish and chill before serving.

Take a can of grapefruit sections and combine these with canned peach halves. Serve them in a glass sherbet dish.

Use a combination of apples, grapefruit slices, and orange slices. Mix these together in a glass sherbet dish and chill before serving.

Use a can of black bing cherries and a can of purple plums. Mix them together, chill, and serve.

A combination of the various types of melons also makes an appetizing and appealing dessert. Use equal balls of honeydew, watermelon, and cantaloupe, mixing them together. If you wish to add a special touch, put a little grenadine on each dish you serve.

A good combination is also made with cantaloupe and bing cherries combined; also with purple plums and cantaloupe.

Honeydew melon combined with diced oranges is a also a good combination.

### Pharoah's Pyramid Exotica

This interesting sweetmeat can be used as an in-between nibbler to keep you from getting too hungry. Combine dates, figs, honey, almonds (chopped), and shredded coconut.

Put the ingredients into a bowl and mix thoroughly. Use about 1 dozen figs, 1 dozen dates, 1 Tbsp. of honey, and about 8 chopped almonds or other nuts. Then mix the shredded coconut with the above ingredients, and shape into pyramids, if you wish to serve them to guests. Put them into your refrigerator until ready to serve as an after-dinner dessert, or you may keep them indefinitely and nibble on them to kill your appetite.

### Bombay Bliss

When serving the previous desserts to guests at lunch or dinner, you can add a touch of the romantic or exotic to your meal by giving these desserts interesting names. The Bombay Bliss is an excellent light dessert, made of fruits, but it looks like a heavy calorie dish, which it is not. The ingredients needed are

Graham crackers

4 ripe bananas

6 peach halves

6 pear halves

1 cup of raisins (soaked until soft)

3 cups of canned blackberries or raspberries

$^{1}/_{4}$ cup shredded coconut

Line a pie tin with a layer of crumbled graham crackers. Put a layer of sliced bananas, a layer of pears, and a layer of peaches over the crackers. Top with blackberries or raspberries, and add raisins. Then sprinkle with coconut, and add a bit of shredded ginger.

To add variety to the above Bombay Bliss you can top the fruit layers with artificial whipped cream, or a cupful of yogurt, or sour cream.

### SHANGHAI APPLE WHIP

2 cups of applesauce

5 egg whites, beaten until thick

1 Tbsp. lemon juice

1 Tbsp. pineapple juice

$^{1}/_{2}$ tsp. ground ginger

1 Tbsp. honey or brown sugar

Beat the egg whites with the honey added, and then put in the applesauce. Add lemon juice and pineapple juice to the mixture, and pour into glasses to chill before serving. Put a touch of ground ginger on top as a garnish.

### ISTANBUL YOGURT—STRAWBERRY DELIGHT

This healthful and tasty dessert adds a few calories to your reducing diet and yet gives great satisfaction to the taste buds. It is also attractive to serve your guests, who will think it exotic and not connect it with dieting at all. You need the following ingredients:

3 cups of strawberries (fresh if possible, if not, frozen will do as well)

$^2/_3$ cup yogurt

$^1/_2$ tsp. vanilla extract

$^1/_2$ tsp. almond extract

4 tsp. honey or artificial sweetener

Mix the yogurt with the washed strawberries, add the vanilla and almond extracts and honey, and mix thoroughly in a bowl. Chill in the refrigerator for an hour or so and serve in glass dishes.

### CREME DE MENTHE BABYLONIAN PINEAPPLE DELIGHT

2 tsp. grated coconut

Several slices of pineapple, canned or fresh

3 Tbsp. creme de menthe

3 tsp. grated ginger

Use chunks or slices of pineapple; place pineapple in a dessert dish, sprinkle creme de menthe over it, and put grated coconut and ginger on top. Garnish with fresh mint leaves, if available. Serve cold.

### TAJ MAHAL FRUIT LOVE CUP

A combination of fruits can be used as a tasty variation to your desserts while dieting or even when on your sustaining diet.

The Taj Mahal Fruit Love Cup uses the following fruits:

3 cups of cantaloupe or honeydew melon balls, or mixed with watermelon balls

3 oranges, cut up into pieces

3 bananas, sliced

1 Tbsp. honey

1 tsp. lemon juice

$^1/_3$ cup grated coconut

Mix the cantaloupe balls, oranges, and bananas with the honey and lemon juice. Then top with grated coconut and chill before serving. To add an exotic touch put a little grenadine on top of each dish.

## MAHARAJAH CANTALOUPE A LA ROYALE

This delicious combination of bananas and cantaloupe is an excellent dessert after a meat or fish dinner.

2 bananas

6 Tbsp. sour cream

2 tsp. honey

1 large cantaloupe

Cut the cantaloupe into 1-inch cubes, after peeling. Mash the 2 bananas in a bowl and add honey and sour cream, mixing them carefully until thoroughly blended. Now put the pieces of cantaloupe into the mixture and toss. Be sure that the sour cream covers all the fruit thoroughly before serving.

## ORIENTAL FRUIT MEDLEY

Use fresh peaches, apricots, and plums for this delicious fruit dessert, if in season. However, you can use canned or frozen fruits if you choose. The following are needed:

4 peaches

4 apricots

4 plums

1 Tbsp. honey

3 ripe or canned plums

3 tsp. lime or lemon juice

3 tsp. pineapple juice

Peel the peaches and apricots if used fresh, and slice them. Mix the honey, lime juice, and pineapple juice together and pour over the fruit.

You can add variety to the above by topping with lemon, orange, pineapple, or raspberry sherbet.

These desserts, being principally fruit, can be used even while you are on the 7-day Oriental reducing diet, without endangering your caloric intake. However, they should be used sparingly, until you have lost your undesired pounds. On your sustaining diet they can be used for the rest of your life and they will satisfy your craving for sweets without giving you the additional calories that would soon put your weight back on again.

# CHAPTER 15

# COUNT YOUR DAILY CALORIES FOR A LIFETIME STAY-SLENDER FOOD PLAN

■ ■ ■

W hat should you know about calories? Is it necessary to count calories for the rest of your life?

There has been a great deal of controversy over this question for many years. Calorie counters say that if one eats food that contains more calories than the body needs for its daily energy requirements those calories will be turned into fat.

There is truth to this statement, for the body can absorb only a certain amount of caloric energy per day. If the body is overloaded with calories it has only one recourse: to convert the unnecessary calories into body fat. Then the fat has to be taken off or there are serious health conditions, as well as unsightly physical conditions to bear.

The consequences of *not* counting calories can readily be seen in the statistics that come out each day on what happens to obese people who have let their calories run away with them. A recent example was that of a famous female singer who weighed 276 pounds and was found dead in her hotel room from a heart condition due to her obesity. Upon performing an autopsy, the physicians found that her heart muscles had begun to turn to fat, impeding their function and leading to a fatal heart attack.

While you are on our Oriental 7-day diet for quick weight loss, it is not necessary to count your calories. The reason for this, as stated earlier, is that you can hardly overeat of the reducing vegetables given in the food plan, and that you can hardly take more rice than the body requires for each day's activity. Rice is very filling and a little goes a long way. Then, when you add meat to the Oriental system of losing weight without hunger, you eat only a small portion each day, and if it is lean meat, this can hardly add enough calories to become a serious problem.

As carbohydrates are practically eliminated in the Oriental diet plan, except for those found in vegetables, there is little concern about starches, sugars, and fats. But when you go on the sustaining diet and eat a balanced meal, including fats, starches, sugars, and proteins, it is obvious that you could soon return to your former state of obesity if you do not restrict your food intake and avoid the high calories that most people take in each meal. The following figures will reveal how few calories the average person needs to remain healthy and slender.

| Sex | Height | Weight | Age | Calories per Day |
|------|--------|--------|-------|------------------|
| Male | 5'10" | 150 | 20–29 | 1750 |
| | | | 30–39 | 1750 |
| | | | 40–49 | 1700 |
| | | | 50–59 | 1650 |
| | | | 60–69 | 1600 |
| | | | 70–79 | 1550 |
| Female | 5'2" | 125 | 20–29 | 1380 |
| | | | 30–39 | 1360 |
| | | | 40–49 | 1340 |
| | | | 50–59 | 1300 |
| | | | 60–69 | 1260 |
| | | | 70–79 | 1230 |

You will notice that the caloric requirements decrease with age. Also, the above caloric requirements are for people who lead a fairly sedentary life, one containing little exercise or physical labor.

If there is a great deal of physical labor and muscle movement then the calorie requirements rise, but a person who is so active seldom puts on weight, no matter how much she eats.

It is the person who gets little exercise and performs no hard work that can get along on the minimum calorie requirements given above.

Children from the age of fourteen to young people of eighteen or more, require slightly more calories, as their activities generally eat up the fat before it is put onto their bodies.

Most weight problems, it is true, are caused by a person taking more calories into her body than she requires for her daily activities. The body has no recourse but to store these unwanted and unneeded calories as fatty tissue.

To show you how serious this problem of obesity is, last year alone the American public spent more than four hundred million dollars on reducing pills, health spas for losing weight, and other methods of weight reduction. Most of these methods achieve the objective of removing unwanted fat, but when the person goes back on her so-called normal diet, she puts the unwanted pounds back again, and the whole vicious cycle has to be repeated again and again.

■ ■ ■

## WHAT YOU SHOULD KNOW ABOUT CALORIES

A calorie is a unit of heat, and has been defined by scientists as the amount of heat required to raise about 2 pounds of water just $1^{\circ}$ centigrade. When you ingest food, calories are supplied that the body requires to combine with oxygen, so it can distribute this digested food to all the body tissues.

To get an idea of the caloric energy released by various foods consider the following: one teaspoon of white sugar provides 16 calories; one teaspoon of olive oil, which is pure fat, releases 36 calories.

Fat produces more calories than protein or carbohydrates. That is one reason why the Oriental reducing plan helps decrease weight quickly, because there is little or no fat content to the foods eaten.

A good way to determine your normal caloric requirements for each day is to find your most desirable weight for your height and age, and then choose the number of calories that fit your requirements.

If you are a sedentary worker, that is, you do not have much physical activity each day, you can determine your required daily calories by multiplying the figure 10 by your normal weight. For example, if you are a man weighing 175 pounds, your average caloric requirements per day would be about 1,750 calories. If you are a woman weighing 125 pounds your ideal caloric intake per day would be 1,250 calories. The moment you absorb more calories than that in your daily food intake, they begin to be stored as excess fat.

However, if you are fairly active in your daily work and move around a good deal, or exercise moderately, such as walking, swimming, or playing golf or tennis, then your caloric requirements would be different. You would multiply your ideal weight by 15, to obtain the number of calories you need per day.

For a 175-pound man then, the caloric intake would now be raised to about 2,625 calories per day. For a woman of 125 pounds, the caloric intake would now be about 1,875 calories per day.

If you do very heavy manual work that requires a great deal of muscular effort and movement, then you would multiply your ideal weight by 20 to obtain your ideal caloric intake. This would raise the caloric requirements for a man weighing 175 pounds to about 3,500 calories per day and for a woman weighing 125 pounds, about 2500 calories per day.

Here are the caloric expenditures per hour for some typical activities, which will help you understand more about your caloric requirements. The following estimates are for a person weighing about 160 pounds.

Riding a bicycle burns up about 200 calories per hour

Boxing requires about 780 calories per hour

Dancing burns up about 260 calories per hour

Washing dishes requires about 70 calories an hour

Eating uses up about 26 calories per hour

Horseback riding, at a trot, requires about 300 calories per hour

Fencing uses up about 500 calories per hour

Piano playing requires about 100 calories per hour

Table tennis requires about 305 calories per hour

Rowing a boat, in competition with others, burns up about 1,120 calories per hour

Running takes up about 500 calories per hour (this is one reason why jogging has become a popular form of exercise)

Swimming takes about 550 calories per hour

Typewriting consumes only about 70 calories an hour

Walking, rapidly, takes 240 calories per hour

Sweeping the floor, with a vacuum cleaner, requires about 200 calories per hour

It can be seen that more strenuous forms of exercise tend to burn up calories more quickly than the milder forms. Very often, when the caloric intake is high, you can burn up those fat-producing extra calories by indulging in some form of exercise that will help melt the fat away.

However, the best thing is to know your calories and figure out how many you need per day, then automatically cut your food intake to those required calories.

Jessie R. was a typical housewife with the usual housework that required about 300 calories an hour for activities such as vacuuming the floor, washing dishes, dusting, shopping, and preparing the meals. However, as she did not work at all these tasks a full eight hours a day (doing her usual housework in about three hours), she spent a great deal of time in watching her favorite romantic stories on TV.

While watching TV Jessie often nibbled on chocolates, and at night, she and her husband had little tidbits, which added considerably to her caloric intake.

When I met Jessie she had gained twenty-five pounds in the three years of her marriage and she couldn't understand why. I checked out her dietary habits and found that she was serving mashed potatoes with the evening meal, with heavy, starchy gravy; at least two times a week she served spaghetti or macaroni (owing to the high cost of meats); and the desserts she served were usually something heavy, like pies, ice creams, or fruits canned in heavy syrup.

The caloric intake was way beyond the normal 1,200 to 1,500 per day that Jessie would ordinarily require to do the work she did. She was consuming at least 2,500 calories a day, and all these extra calories were being rapidly turned into fatty deposits on her hips and stomach.

It was necessary for Jessie to cut down on her calories. She was able to get rid of the twenty-five extra pounds within three weeks on the Oriental diet, and then she went on the sustaining diet, allowing herself about 1,500 calories a day for her normal routine. She seemed to hold her weight down to normal in the ensuing months.

When you have determined the number of calories you require for your particular age and activities for any given day, you can determine each day's caloric intake and then try to approximate it. If you find yourself putting on a few extra pounds, or you carelessly eat too many carbohydrate and starchy foods, cut down on your fat calories for a few days. Then when you are back to your normal weight, you can resume your normal diet.

It is perfectly natural for you to vary five pounds one way or the other in your monthly weight. Do not be alarmed at these fluctuations, but if you should go over the five-pound mark, immediately start your Oriental diet, eating more brown rice and vegetables, and fewer starches and carbohydrates. In one week you will shed the extra pounds without effort.

I have calculated the caloric contents of all the major foods that you may eat in the future, and these appear in the Appendix of this book. Consult this list to find out the approximate calories that your general diet contains. Then figure out your menu according to this list so you never go beyond your normal caloric intake for each day.

Very soon you will find yourself so expert in judging your caloric intake that you will automatically form the habit of selecting the right foods for your particular age and weight.

In the following chapter we shall learn some of the Oriental techniques for maintaining a good mental attitude through philosophy and daily meditation. This will help you develop the balance you need to keep you in perfect mental, emotional, and physical health.

# CHAPTER 16

# ADD YOGA POWER
# TO YOUR ORIENTAL
# SYSTEM OF
# REDUCING
# WITHOUT HUNGER

**M**illions of people throughout the world today are using yoga power to help them achieve mastery of their minds and bodies.

It is vitally important in our Oriental system of reducing without hunger to utilize this regimen of control, to make it easier for you to keep weight off, as well as to give you the mental power to stay on your reducing diet until you have achieved the desired results.

What does the word yoga mean? It literally means to be yoked to a higher power than the ordinary conscious mind we all possess. It admits of a system of mental and physical control that enlists the aid of higher forces within the mind, which psychologists call the subconscious and superconscious minds.

Many Yogis, using mind control alone, have regulated the metabolism of their bodies so that the body threw off many of the foods that produce fat deposits.

Now through scientific research in what is called alpha biofeedback training, the mind is shown to release brainwaves that are called alpha, theta, and beta. In each of these states of brainwave activity, produced by a high degree of concentration called meditation, the person trying to control his mind and body is able to regulate such functions as heart action, digestion, blood pressure, and other vital functions of the body, including the metabolic processes that determine what foods the body shall absorb and what foods it shall throw off.

By using yoga meditation during your times of reducing you will avoid the nervousness, fatigue, and stress that often come to people who try to reduce or change their food habits in any way. As you will be adopting a new food plan for the rest of your life after losing the undesired pounds, it is vitally important that you know how to use yoga power to avoid the side effects that come from dieting or maintaining the lifetime sustaining diet.

Ella D., a woman who came to me for help in solving her weight problem, weighed 185 pounds. She was very short, and her normal weight should have been 120, for her age and height. She had tried various diets to lose weight but found that she could not stay on them for more than a few days at a time. She said, "I get highly tense and nervous when I am dieting. I suppose I use food as an outlet for my emotional frustrations and problems at home."

It was then that she told me the real reason for seeking me out: she and her husband had not been getting along well for several months. As she gained weight he had lost interest in her sexually. She was forty-six years of age, and she said her husband no longer found her sexually appealing. She suspected he was seeing another woman, for he was forty-eight and she knew that he should still be at the peak of his sexual vigor.

I knew that this woman needed more than a weight-losing regimen to solve her emotional problems. She needed a life philosophy that would make it easier for her to diet and also to solve her marital problems after she lost her unwanted pounds.

It was very difficult for this woman to remain on the Oriental diet, for she felt a craving for sweets constantly. I gave her one dessert a day that she could indulge in without adding too many extra calories, and then I made her practice various states of meditation to gain control of her mind and her nerves.

It was amazing to see the change that came over this woman. By the time she had lost her weight, which took her three months of real work, she had become so agreeable and free from tension that her husband began to show romantic interest again, and told her she was like the girl he had married years before. In fact, when she had finally gotten down to her 120 pounds, she had to have a complete new wardrobe, which he gladly bought for her and as an extra bonus, he surprised her by taking her to Hawaii for a second honeymoon!

■ ■ ■

## ORIENTAL REGIMEN FOR KEEPING YOUR WEIGHT DOWN

**1.** Adopt a philosophy of peace and quiescence in your everyday life. See the events in the outer world as a panorama that is being projected on a giant motion picture screen. View it with interest but not with alarm. Do not let yourself react to the violence, confusion, and discord that is in the outer world. View it all as a spectator—do not react with tension, alarm, nervousness, and excitability. The Buddha is pictured throughout the Orient as a calm figure, with imperturbable features that reflect only peace and quiet.

The reason this is vitally important in helping you control your body and its metabolism it that when you are quiet and calm within, your body's metabolism is favorably affected. Your heart action will be normal, your blood pressure will remain perfect, and your body will respond with the perfect functioning of all your glands and other organs.

**2.** With the previous exercise to maintain your peace and quiet, combine the breathing techniques used for achieving tranquillity. Oxygen is the perfect tranquilizer. You breathe every moment, because this is one of the most important functions of the body for maintaining life. It is more important than food or water. You can live for days without food, as the body feeds on its own fat when it is deprived of food; you can live for three or four days without water; but you cannot live more than a few moments without air. This is why yogis practice breathing techniques frequently, which helps the body burn up the foods that have been ingested and distribute them through the bloodstream to build the body cells.

The breathing to practice for achieving this state of calmness is practiced in hatha yoga, which is for the maintenance of the body's strength, health, and energy. Breathe in to the count of four; hold the breath to the count of four, and then breathe out to the count of four. Do this five to ten times, at least three times a day, and flush out the fatigue acids, toxins, and other chemical wastes that gather in the bloodstream.

This is the tranquilizing breath of yoga, which helps soothe the nerves and which causes the heart action to be normal, the metabolism to be perfect, and the glands to operate normally.

How a Man Used Tranquilizing Breath to Overcome a Weight Problem and Bad Temper. It is a well-known fact that oxygen intake is nature's way of oxidizing the body and helping the processes of metabolism and absorption of the foods eaten.

When the mind is constantly disturbed and the emotions get out of control, it has a drastic effect on the metabolism as well as on the glandular system.

Robert W. was a two hundred pound executive in a large manufacturing plant. He not only had high blood pressure and symptoms of a serious heart ailment, but his temper flared frequently, and he was highly nervous, tense, and anxious about the future. All these things contributed to his tendency to overeat and to keep gaining weight.

Robert was thoroughly checked by his family doctor, who told him he must lose weight if he wanted to avoid serious health complications. The man came into our lecture work, forced by his wife, who had been a former member, and she got him on the Oriental reducing diet. But with his temper, impatience, and tendency to disbelieve anything connected with meditation, yoga, and other forms of philosophy, he simply could not see himself becoming a student of philosophy.

When he began to see the fat melting away, however, he changed his mind and began to come to regular classes on meditation. He started the tranquilizing breath with meditation and soon had lowered his blood pressure to near normal. He gained such control of his mind that his temper outbursts were completely overcome. He is now on the way to perfect health.

**3.** When you awaken in the morning adopt your philosophy for the entire day. View the world as being a wonderful place in which to live. Thank God for another day of life, and then dedicate your mind, body, and soul to your creator. A good meditation to achieve this oneness with creative life energy is the following:

*I thank God for another day of life. I now dedicate my mind to the reception of inspirational ideas for the betterment of the world. I dedicate my breath as a living prayer to God. Each time I breathe I direct my breath to be a living prayer to the greater glory of God. I dedicate my body as a chalice to the flow of God's life power, so I may be strong and healthy and better serve Him and humanity.*

*I direct my body and all its functions to operate at peak efficiency, so I shall be strong, healthy, and have youthful vitality throughout my natural life span.*

I learned of this dedication ceremony from a Tibetan monk I once met in the northern part of India, within view of the Himalayas. He was resting under a tree at noontime, and he was turning a prayer wheel. I stopped to photograph him, and I asked him what he was doing. He then explained that every time his prayer wheel turned, a hundred prayers, attached to the wheel, ascended to the celestial heights. Then he told me how to be in perpetual touch with the cosmic life energy that gives us perfect power for every day's living. By dedicating our mind, body, and soul to God each day when we awaken, we are in touch with the source of life and power. The word yoga literally means to be yoked to the power that created us and that sustains us.

**4.** Adopt the Oriental attitude that your soul will live forever and that there is no need for the hustle and bustle that catches us up and wears us down. One of the reasons why so many millions of people in this country are sick mentally and physically is that they live under pressure. The stresses of modern living, with its daily shocks and tragedies, tend to upset the emotional balance of the average person. This in turn affects the nervous system and the heart, blood pressure, metabolism, and other vital functions of the body, including the secretions of the glands. When a person is in a state of perpetual shock, her nervous reactions are such that they release adrenaline into the blood stream. This in turn accelerates the heart and blood pressure, causing it to become erratic. A chemical known as epinephrine is released into the bloodstream, and can poison the body and paralyze its normal functions. Most people are in a perpetual state of shock from the rapidly shifting, tragic scene of events in the outer world, and they react so emotionally that their bodies never recover from these recurring shocks.

Oriental philosophy will help you maintain a state of calm and to adjust to the changing scene with inner poise and equanimity.

**5.** Repeat the following tranquilizing statements several times a day when you are faced with emotional turmoil.

> *My mind is like a peaceful lake without a ripple on the surface. I am peaceful and calm and no outer winds of misfortune can disturb the center of my being where there is only calm and tranquillity.*
>
> *I ascend to the spiritual mountain top where I rise above the world of war, disaster, sickness, and death. On this mountain peak I see into the illimitable vistas of eternity. I rise above my problems into a stratosphere of spiritual poise and power. I look up at the perpetual glory of God's infinite universe and remove myself from the scenes of turbulence and tragedy.*

■ ■ ■

## MEDITATION SAVES A WOMAN FROM COMPLETE COLLAPSE

Mrs. Sadie J. had been a widow for years, but her grief at losing her husband of thirty years was so overwhelming that she lost all desire to live. She was brought to me by her oldest son, who said they had taken their mother to a psychiatrist to help her overcome her melancholy. The therapy had not helped, and they thought my work might assist her in regaining her emotional balance.

Mrs. J. was only ten pounds overweight, and this she was able to lose in one week on the Oriental diet, but I realized that she had to have a sustaining philosophy to keep her alive and to give her a future goal towards which she could aspire.

I showed Mrs. J. how to go into daily meditation, using the alpha brainwave techniques (what is known as hatha yoga in India), and she began to respond from the very first day. I told her to withdraw into her beautiful memories of the happy, romantic thirty years she had spent with her perfect husband and three times daily, to do these meditations. I did not urge her, as some therapists might have, to forget the past and live for the future, for as a student of mysticism, I realized that the dream is often more real than reality. By going back over her memory paths of the joyous years with her husband, she was keeping alive the memory and easing the pain of his death. In two months' time she was ready to begin her mental journey into the future. She was soon so strong mentally and emotionally that she could face going out socially once more. Soon she was attending senior dances and having a joyous time. Her son reported to me six months later that his mother had met a retired doctor who had a beautiful home in the country and had asked her to marry him! Whether she does or does not marry, Mrs. J. is on the way to a happy, zestful life because she discovered the secret strength that can come when a person becomes spiritually oriented by a deep, abiding faith and meditation.

■ ■ ■

## HUMANS ARE THREE-DIMENSIONAL BEINGS

Humans operate on three planes of consciousness: they are mental, physical, and spiritual. Only when you learn to operate on these three planes of consciousness do you achieve perfect balance between the mind, body, and soul.

In attempting any system of dieting, realize that "Man shall not live by bread alone." It is necessary that you have an adequate spiritual philosophy to sustain you and give you the balance that all great mystics have told us is essential to healthy, happy, and successful living.

Now you have the keys that are needed to open the doors of consciousness. The sustaining diet that will keep you healthy and well nourished should be followed all the days of your life.

Do not worry if you put on a few extra pounds occasionally. Check your weight daily on the bathroom scale, and the moment the weight goes up five or six pounds, go right back on the Oriental quick weight-loss diet. By doing so, you can keep that weight down without effort in the future.

Keep your mind and emotions under control, through the Oriental philosophy we have given in this book, and use meditation and prayer daily to keep your soul attuned to the spiritual power of the universe.

As you journey into the future, new and exciting experiences await you! You have learned how to live under the natural laws of the universe, using natural foods that God gave humans to sustain them in perfect health. With your good health and normal weight, you will be ready for the greatest adventures of your life, with perfect health and energy to sustain you for a hundred years or more of zestful, joyous living!

# THE CALORIC VALUES OF CERTAIN FOODS

T
he following list of foods and their caloric content must be understood to be approximate, for it is difficult to evaluate the exact caloric content of food. However, most nutritional experts come close to agreement on the number of calories in most basic foods.

■ ■ ■

---

# MEATS

(Calories are estimated for a four-ounce serving.)

|  | CALORIES |
|---|---|
| *Beef* | |
| Hamburger, broiled and fat removed | 210 |
| Beef, boiled | 235 |
| Filet mignon | 200 |
| Liver, broiled | 165 |
| Pot roast | 245 |
| Corned beef | 260 |
| Beef heart, baked | 125 |
| Prime rib of beef, roasted | 190 |
| Sirloin steak | 210 |
| Sweetbreads, broiled | 190 |
| Kidneys, stewed | 190 |
| Tripe, stewed | 118 |
| Beef tongue, boiled | 310 |
| Round steak, broiled | 180 |
| Calf brains | 145 |
| | |
| *Chicken* | |
| Broiled | 150 |
| Boiled | 240 |
| Creamed ($^1/_2$ cup) | 210 |
| Breast, roasted | 165 |
| Leg, roasted | 210 |
| | |
| *Duck* | |
| Roasted | 360 |
| | |
| *Goose* | |
| Roasted | 375 |

CALORIES

*Lamb*

| | |
|---|---|
| Chops | 230 |
| Leg, roasted | 215 |
| Mutton chops | 210 |
| Mutton, boiled | 205 |
| Leg of mutton, roasted | 355 |

*Pork*

| | |
|---|---|
| Chops, broiled | 220 |
| Ham, baked | 180 |
| Ham, deviled (1 Tbsp.) | 85 |
| Ham, smoked | 180 |
| Loin of pork, roasted | 210 |
| Sausage, fried | 400 |
| Bacon, crisp, broiled (4 strips) | 120 |

*Sausage*

| | |
|---|---|
| Bologna | 255 |
| Liverwurst | 285 |
| Pork (1 normal length) | 90 |
| Salami | 525 |
| Frankfurter (1 average) | 145 |

*Turkey*

| | |
|---|---|
| Breast, roasted | 215 |
| Dark meat | 225 |

*Veal*

| | |
|---|---|
| Cutlets, broiled | 180 |
| Cutlets, fried | 245 |
| Leg of veal, roasted | 180 |

■ ■ ■

## FISH AND SEAFOOD

|  | CALORIES |
|---|---|
| *Abalone broiled* (3 1/2 oz.) | 108 |
| *Bass, broiled or baked* (4 oz.) | 180 |
| *Bluefish, broiled or baked* (4 oz.) | 180 |
| *Caviar* (2 Tbsp.) | 70 |
| *Clams* | |
| Canned (3 oz.) | 44 |
| Cherrystone (4 oz.) | 90 |
| Littleneck (4 oz.) | 90 |
| Steamed (6—with butter | 140 |
| *Cod* (4 oz.) | 100 |
| Balls (small, 2) | 75 |
| Baked (1 med.-sized) | 125 |
| Dry (1 oz.) | 105 |
| Salted (4 oz.) | 140 |
| Steak (1 med. piece) | 100 |
| *Crab* | |
| Cracked (1 med.-sized) | 95 |
| Hard-shell (4 oz.) | 95 |
| Soft-shell (4 oz.) | 90 |
| *Finnan Haddie* (4 oz.) | 100 |
| Smoked (4 oz.) | 100 |

| | |
|---|---|
| *Flounder* (4 oz.) | 75 |
| *Gefilte fish* (4 oz.) | 75 |
| *Haddock* (1 fillet) | 160 |
|     Creamed (4 oz.) | 150 |
|     Fried | 165 |
| *Halibut, broiled* (4 oz.) | 135 |
| *Herring* (4 oz.) | 215 |
|     Pickled | 105 |
|     Pickled, with sour cream | 250 |
|     Smoked | 245 |
| *Lobster* | |
|     Baked or broiled (1 average size) | 125 |
|     Creamed (4 oz.) | 155 |
|     With butter | 300 |
|     Cocktail (1 average) | 80 |
|         $1/_2$ cup meat with sauce | 100 |
|         $1/_2$ cup meat with lemon | 75 |
|         $1/_2$ cup meat with mayonnaise | 95 |
|     Newburgh ($1/_2$ cup.) | 125 |
|     Thermador (1 lobster) | 210 |
| *Oysters* | |
|     Fried (3 large pieces) | 250 |
|     Raw (4 oz.) | 100 |
|     Stewed (8 oz. cup) | 250 |
|     Scalloped (6) | 250 |
|     Stew, $1/_2$ cream (8 oz.) | 200 |

<small>CALORIES</small>

| | |
|---|---|
| *Porgy* (4 oz.) | 110 |
| *Red fish* (4 oz.) | 100 |
| *Red snapper* (4 oz.) | 95 |

*Salmon*

| | |
|---|---|
| Baked or broiled (medium portion) | 205 |
| Chinook (4 oz.) | 175 |
| Smoked (4 oz.) | 285 |

*Sardines*

| | |
|---|---|
| Without oil (3 oz.) | 180 |
| With oil (3 oz.) | 288 |
| With tomato sauce (3 oz.) | 185 |

*Scallops*

| | |
|---|---|
| Broiled (4 oz.) | 175 |
| Fried (4 oz.—3 large pieces) | 295 |

| | |
|---|---|
| *Seafood au gratin* ($^1/_2$ cup) | 300 |

| | |
|---|---|
| *Shad* (4 oz.) | 190 |
| Roe (2 oz.) | 100 |

*Shrimp*

| | |
|---|---|
| Canned (3 oz.) | 110 |
| Fresh (6 med.) | 75 |
| Fried (6 med.) | 100 |

CALORIES

*Shrimp* (cont'd)

| | |
|---|---|
| Cocktail ($^1/_3$ cup with sauce) | 85 |
| Creole ( 6 shrimp with sauce) | 160 |

*Smelt*

| | |
|---|---|
| Fried with butter (2–3) | 150 |

*Sole*

| | |
|---|---|
| Fillet (4 oz.) | 100 |
| Sautéed (4 oz.) | 236 |

*Squid*

| | |
|---|---|
| Dried (4 oz.) | 305 |

*Smoked sturgeon* (3 oz.)     110

*Sword fish* (1 piece)     223

*Trout*

| | |
|---|---|
| Brook trout (4 oz.) | 50 |
| Smoked (3 oz.) | 100 |

*Tuna*

| | |
|---|---|
| Canned, drained (3 oz.) | 175 |
| Canned, with oil (3 oz.) | 245 |
| Creamed (4 oz.) | 270 |
| Fresh (3 oz.) | 150 |
| Smoked (3 oz.) | 130 |
| Casserole (1 average portion, with noodles) | 300 |

■ ■ ■

## VEGETABLES

|  | CALORIES |
|---|---|
| *Artichokes* | |
| Canned hearts (5) | 37 |
| Jerusalem (4 small) | 78 |
| Bottoms (1 normal) | 30 |
| | |
| *Asparagus* | |
| Cooked stalks (6) | 22 |
| Cut spears ($^3/_4$ cup) | 45 |
| Canned (6 spears) | 22 |
| Frozen (6 spears) | 22 |
| | |
| *Bamboo shoots* (4 oz.) | 30 |
| | |
| Beans | |
| Baked, with pork, brown sugar, or molasses (1 cup) | 325 |
| Canned baked (1 cup) | 325 |
| Tomato sauce (1 cup | 295 |
| Green beans, cooked (1 cup) | 27 |
| Green beans, canned ($^3/_4$ cup) | 50 |
| Kidney beans (7 Tbsp.) | 180 |
| Lima beans ($^1/_2$ cup cooked) | 180 |
| Lima beans, canned (1 cup) | 175 |
| Lima beans, frozen (4 oz.) | 130 |
| | |
| *Bean sprouts* (1 cup) | 27 |

CALORIES

*Beets*

    Greens ($1/_2$ cup cooked)     40
    Raw (2 medium)     105
    Cooked ($1/_2$ cup)     55
    Canned ($1/_2$ cup)     60
    Pickled (1 cup)     55

*Broccoli*

    Cooked (1 cup)     44
    Frozen (2–3 spears)     20

*Brussels Sprouts, cooked* (1 cup)     44

*Cabbage*

    Shredded (1 cup)     24
    Chinese (1 cup)     15

*Carrots*

    Raw (1)     21
    Raw, grated (1 cup)     45
    Cooked (1 cup)     44
    Canned (1 cup)     44

*Cauliflower*

    Buds (1 cup)     25
    Cooked (1 cup)     30
    Frozen (1 cup)     35

CALORIES

| | |
|---|---:|
| *Celery* (1 large stalk) | 7 |
| Cooked (1 cup) | 18 |
| *Chard leaves and stalks, cooked* (1 cup) | 30 |
| *Chives, chopped* (4 oz.) | 30 |
| *Chicory* (5–6 leaves) | 18 |
| *Collards* (1 cup) | 76 |
| *Coriander* (4 oz.) | 140 |
| *Corn* (1 ear) | 150 |
| Canned with liquid (1 cup | 170 |
| Fritters (1) | 50 |
| *Cucumbers* (1 med. | 12 |
| *Dandelion greens, cooked* ($^3/_4$ cup) | 75 |
| *Eggplant* ($^1/_2$ cup) | 52 |
| *Endive* (10 leaves) | 6 |
| *Escarole* (2 large leaves) | 6 |
| *Fennel* (1 cup) | 8 |
| *Garlic* (1 clove) | 5 |
| *Ginger root* (4 oz.) | 55 |

CALORIES

| | |
|---|---|
| *Hominy grits, cooked* ($^1/_2$ cup) | 65 |
| *Horseradish* (1 Tbsp.) | 12 |
| *Kale, cooked* ($^1/_2$ cup) | 55 |
| *Kohlrabi, cooked* (8 oz.) | 72 |
| *Leeks* (3 med.) | 42 |
| *Lentils* ($^3/_4$ cup) | 315 |
| *Lettuce* (1 head) | 68 |
| *Lotus root* ($^2/_3$ segment) | 49 |

*Mushrooms*
| | |
|---|---|
| Fresh ( 8 oz.—sliced) | 20 |
| Sautéed (7 small) | 60 |
| Canned (1 cup with liquid) | 28 |

| | |
|---|---|
| *Mustard greens, cooked* (1 cup) | 30 |
| *Mustard, dry* (1 tsp.) | 10 |
| *Okra, cooked* ($^1/_2$ cup) | 20 |

*Olives*
| | |
|---|---|
| Green (10 large) | 105 |
| Ripe or black (10 large) | 135 |
| Stuffed (5 large) | 55 |

CALORIES

*Onions*

| | |
|---|---:|
| Raw (1 med.) | 49 |
| Cooked (1 cup) | 79 |
| Green onions (6 small) | 23 |
| Scalloped ($^1/_2$ cup) | 70 |
| Fried ($^1/_2$ cup) | 162 |
| Creamed ($^1/_2$ cup) | 109 |

| | |
|---|---:|
| *Parsnips, cooked* ($^1/_2$ cup) | 47 |
| Raw (4 oz.) | 78 |

*Peas*

| | |
|---|---:|
| Black-eyed (1 cup) | 150 |
| Fresh, cooked (1 cup | 111 |
| Canned with liquid (1 cup) | 168 |
| Frozen ($^1/_2$ cup) | 14 |
| Split (1 cup) | 14 |
| Fresh garden peas, shelled (4 oz.) | 90 |

*Peppers*

| | |
|---|---:|
| Green (1 medium) | 16 |
| Stuffed (1 medium) | 185 |
| Red, dried (1 Tbsp.) | 52 |
| Fresh (1 med.) | 28 |
| Cooked (1 med.) | 17 |

*Pickles*

| | |
|---|---:|
| Chow chow (4 pcs.) | 7 |
| Cucumber (4 slices) | 20 |
| Dill (1 med.) | 15 |
| Sweet (1 large) | 22 |
| Sour (1 large) | 15 |
| Sweet mixed relish with mustard (1 Tbsp.) | 16 |
| Sweet mixed relish (1 Tbsp.) | 14 |

CALORIES

| | |
|---|---|
| *Pimento* (1 med. canned) | 10 |
| *Potato chips* (10) | 108 |

*Potatoes*

| | |
|---|---|
| Au gratin (4 oz.) | 250 |
| Baked or boiled (1 med.) | 100 |
| Creamed (3–4 small) | 130 |
| French-fried (10 pieces) | 157 |
| Hash brown (1 cup) | 470 |
| Frozen french fried (10 pieces) | 148 |
| Mashed, with milk ($^1/_2$ cup) | 80 |
| Mashed, with butter ($^1/_2$ cup) | 120 |
| Baked, unpeeled (1 med.) | 102 |
| Baked, peeled (1 med.) | 97 |
| Boiled, peeled (1 medium) | 180 |
| Boiled, unpeeled (1 lb.) | 359 |

| | |
|---|---|
| *Pumpkin* (4 oz.) | 105 |
| *Radishes* (4 small) | 7 |
| *Rice, cooked* (8 oz. cup) | 205 |
| *Sauerkraut* ($^1/_4$ cup drained) | 27 |
| *Scallions* (4 med.) | 8 |
| *Soybeans* ($^1/_2$ cup) | 120 |
| *Soybean sprouts* (1 cup) | 60 |

*Spinach*

| | |
|---|---|
| Cooked (1 cup) | 46 |
| Raw ($1/_2$ lb.) | 44 |
| Canned (1 cup) | 46 |

*Squash*

| | |
|---|---|
| Hubbard or winter, baked ($1/_2$ cup) | 50 |
| Summer squash, boiled ($1/_2$ cup) | 20 |

*String beans* ($1/_2$ cup)    25

*Sweet Potatoes*

| | |
|---|---|
| Baked (1 | 140 |
| Candied (1 small) | 314 |
| Boiled (1 lb.) | 560 |

*Tomatoes*

| | |
|---|---|
| Canned (8 oz. cup) | 46 |
| Fresh (1 med.) | 30 |
| Stewed (9 oz.) | 50 |

| | |
|---|---|
| *Turnips, tops* ($1/_2$ cup) | 49 |
| Cooked ($1/_2$ cup) | 22 |

*Watercress* (1 lb.)    180

*Watercress* (10 pcs.)    2

*Yams*

| | |
|---|---|
| Cooked (1 cup) | 260 |
| Baked (1 cup) | 183 |
| Candied (1 small) | 314 |

*Zucchini* ($1/_2$ cup)    23

■ ■ ■

## FRUITS

|  | CALORIES |
|---|---|
| *Apple, raw* (1 med.) | 85 |
| Baked with sugar | 200 |
| Cooked, unsweetened | 120 |
| Dried, cooked, and sweetened ($^1/_4$ cup) | 102 |
| *Applesauce* | |
| Canned, sweetened (8 oz.) | 260 |
| Unsweetened (8 oz.) | 120 |
| *Apricots* | |
| Canned in syrup (4 med.) | 97 |
| Dried, cooked, unsweetened ($^1/_2$ cup) | 130 |
| Stewed (8 oz.) | 400 |
| *Avocado* ($^1/_2$) | 280 |
| *Bananas* (1 large) | 120 |
| Fried (1 med.) | 140 |
| *Blackberries, fresh* (1 cup) | 82 |
| Canned with syrup (8 oz. cup) | 245 |
| Frozen, sweetened (1 cup) | 160 |
| *Blueberries, fresh* (1 cup) | 85 |
| Canned with syrup (8 oz.) | 245 |
| Frozen, sweetened (1 cup) | 160 |

CALORIES

*Boysenberries*

| | |
|---|---|
| Frozen, sweetened (1 cup) | 160 |
| Frozen, unsweetened (1 cup) | 70 |

*Cantaloupe* ($^1/_2$ med. size)    37

*Casaba melon* (1 wedge)    52

*Cherries, fresh* (1 cup)    64
    Canned (8 oz. cup)    94

*Coconut* (1 med. piece)    161
    Shredded, sweetened (8 oz. cup)    349

*Cranberries* (8 oz.)    54
    Sauce, sweetened (8 oz.)    549

*Dates* (3–4)    100

*Figs* (2–3)    90
    Canned with syrup (3 figs)    130
    Dried figs (1 large)    57

*Fruit cocktail, canned* (6 oz.)    110

*Gooseberries* (8 oz.)    60

*Grapes* (4 oz.)    80
    Thompson seedless (8 oz.)    150

CALORIES

| | |
|---|---|
| *Grapefruit* ($^1/_2$ large) | 104 |
| Canned, sweetened (8 oz.) | 180 |
| Canned, unsweetened (8 oz.) | 90 |
| *Honeydew melon* (1 med. wedge) | 49 |
| *Lemon* (1 med.) | 40 |
| *Loganberries* ($^2/_3$ cup) | 70 |
| Canned, sweetened (8 oz.) | 104 |
| *Mangoes* (1 med.) | 48 |
| *Nectarine* (1 med.) | 38 |
| *Oranges* | |
| Large | 106 |
| Medium | 70 |
| *Papaya, fresh* (8 oz.) | 71 |
| *Passion fruit* (4 oz.) | 100 |
| *Peach* (1 med.) | 77 |
| Canned, with syrup (8 oz.) | 174 |
| *Pears* (1 med.) | 95 |
| Canned, with syrup (2 halves) | 90 |

| | CALORIES |
|---|---:|
| *Persian melon* (1 med. wedge) | 52 |
| *Persimmons* (8 oz. med.) | 250 |
| *Pineapple, fresh* (1 slice med.) | 44 |
| Canned, syrup (1 large slice) | 95 |
| Frozen (4 oz.) | 118 |
| *Plums, fresh* (8 oz) | 94 |
| Canned (8 oz.) | 210 |
| *Prunes, dried* (1 small) | 14 |
| Cooked, no sugar (8 oz.) | 200 |
| Cooked, with sugar (8 oz.) | 320 |
| *Raisins, dried* (1 Tbsp.) | 26 |
| Cooked, with sugar (8 oz.) | 572 |
| *Raspberries, red, fresh* (8 oz.) | 70 |
| Frozen (3 oz.) | 126 |
| *Rhubarb* (8 oz.) | 19 |
| *Strawberries* (8 oz. cup) | 54 |
| Frozen (3 oz.) | 90 |
| Fresh (5 large) | 25 |
| *Watermelon* ($1/_2$ slice) | 45 |
| 1 med. wedge | 100 |
| Balls or cubes ($1/_2$ cup) | 35 |

■ ■ ■

## ICE CREAM

|  | CALORIES |
|---|---|
| Banana (1 scoop) | 292 |
| Banana split (regular size) | 1,165 |
| Butter pecan (1 scoop) | 297 |
| Chocolate (1 scoop) | 298 |
| Chocolate chip (1 scoop) | 298 |
| Chocolate malted milk (regular size) | 305 |
| with ice cream | 600 |
| Chocolate sundae (regular) | 318 |
| Fudge sundae | 330 |
| Lemon ice | 116 |
| Peach (1 scoop) | 295 |
| Pineapple (1 scoop) | 250 |
| Vanilla (fountain size) | 420 |

■ ■ ■

## FATS

|  | CALORIES |
|---|---|
| Bacon fat (1 Tbsp.) | 100 |
| Beef drippings (1 Tbsp.) | 50 |
| Butter, salted (1 Tbsp.) | 100 |
| Sweet (1 Tbsp.) | 100 |
| Chicken fat (1 Tbsp.) | 150 |
| Cooking fat (1 Tbsp.) | 110 |
| Corn oil (1 Tbsp.) | 100 |
| Cottonseed oil (1 Tbsp.) | 100 |
| Crisco (1 Tbsp.) | 110 |
| Lard (8 oz. cup) | 1,984 |
| Olive oil (1 Tbsp.) | 125 |

|  | CALORIES |
|---|---|
| Peanut butter (1 Tbsp.) | 93 |
| Peanut oil (1 Tbsp.) | 118 |
| Salad and cooking oil (1 Tbsp.) | 124 |
| Vegetable oil (1 Tbsp.) | 110 |

■ ■ ■

## FLOURS

|  | CALORIES |
|---|---|
| Barley (8 oz.) | 420 |
| Buckwheat (8 oz.) | 340 |
| Cornmeal (8 oz.) | 120 |
| Corn soya (8 oz.) | 125 |
| Cornstarch (1 Tbsp.) | 37 |
| Soybean (8 oz.) | 285 |
| Whole wheat (8 oz.) | 401 |
| Wheat germ (8 oz.) | 423 |

Using this list of foods and their caloric content, you can easily make up your own daily sustaining diet, keeping within the calorie count essential for your age and normal weight. If you binge occasionally and begin to put on those unwanted pounds, go back to your Oriental reducing diet, and then eat the low-calorie foods in this list that will permit you to retain your normal weight and at the same time keep you from being fatigued.

# PRODUCT INFORMATION

■ ■ ■

## WAKUNAGA OF AMERICA CO., LTD.

The following products mentioned toward the end of Chapter 10 are a critical part of the Oriental 7-Day Quick Weight-Off Diet. They are *the best* supplements in America today for effective weight loss and consistent management of the desired body weight once it is achieved. They are readily available in most health food stores nationwide.

> Kyo-Green Powdered Drink Mix
> Kyolic Aged Garlic Extract Super Formula 106
> Kyolic Aged Garlic Extract Dietary Supplement Formula 105
> Premium Kyolic-EPA
> Liquid Kyolic Aged Garlic Extract
> Gingko Biloba Plus
> Kyo-Dophilus

For more information, please contact:

Wakunaga of America Co., Ltd.
23501 Madero
Mission Viejo, CA 92691
1-800-421-2998
1-800-544-5800 (Calif. only)
1-714-458-2764 fax
Telex: 664226 KYOLIC TRNC

■ ■ ■

## VITA-MIX CORPORATION

Some of the recipes cited within this book call for the use of a food blender. The finest unit in America that we know of is the Vita-Mix Total Nutrition Center. It is inexpensive, simple to operate, and easy to clean. Its superb quality is fully backed with a guarantee. For more information, please write or call:

Vita-Mix Corporation
8615 Usher Road
Cleveland, OH 44138
1-800-VITAMIX (800-848-2649)

# INDEX

pg.
49-51, 140
126, 167-199